Tiandidao
Qigong & Baduanjin
Taoist Health & Fitness Exercises

by
Professor Mike Symonds.

Taoist Qigong covers a broad spectrum of exercise that lies between keeping fit and healthy at one end and medical practice at the other. This book introduces and covers the safe basics.

Published by:
Life Force Books
www.Life-Force-Publishing.co.uk

ISBN: 0-9542932-2-3
ISBN (13): 978-0-9542932-2-2
EAN: 9780954293222

©Copyright and all International rights reserved 'Life Force Books' publications and T'ien Ti Tao Academy and Professor Mike Symonds all International rights reserved. No part of this publication may be reproduced in any form or by any means whatsoever be it graphic, electronic, or mechanical, including photocopying, recording, taping or information storage and retrieval systems - without the prior permission in writing of the author and International copyright owner. The author, publishers and printers or their representatives make no claims, express or implied, with regard to the accuracy of the information contained within this book and cannot accept any legal responsibility for any errors or omissions.

First Edition (Paperback) 2009
Life Force publishing.

DEDICATIONS AND SINCERE THANKS

Dedicated to my lovely daughters, Kristie, Jane & Rebecca whom I hope will all learn, benefit from this and continue to spread the goodness of Tao.

*

WITH SINCERE THANKS AND GRATITUDE TO:
The Late Grandmaster C. Chee Soo
All the "Tao Science" Developers, past and present.
Shih-fu Terry Windsor for his editing work.

*

The Taoist Arts are not about personal gain,
Although we have to live.
The arts concern the quality of life,
And when we learn we give.

*

IMPORTANT READER NOTICE:

This book replaces the original 'Pa T'uan Chin Qigong' book published in the late 1980's as a Comb-bound A4 (C4) book intended for students and this book adds more depth and answers to Qigong in general following many requests to "demystify" this ancient Art.

Qigong and general Chinese health and fitness exercises are a wonderful thing and as often as not associated with healing or maintaining good health. However, this book is *not* intended as a set of instructions to follow as a D.I.Y. (Do It Yourself) manual, but is aimed at furthering the knowledge of experienced instructors and their advancing students.

If you, dear reader, have any health problems, or suspect that you are not "100%", then arrange to go see a health specialist before taking up any form of exercise or therapy. Especially do not attempt or practice Qigong or similar Arts if you have a high temperature, low metabolic rate, high blood pressure, back problems (correct posture advice needed) or other debilitating dis-eases: Qigong, like Taijiquan, can help many of the above dis-eases (dis-ease – to be not at ease) but it is essential to get proper diagnosis from an expert; not necessarily a GP (General Practitioner).

CONTENTS	Page No.
Introduction	01
What is Ch'i Kung (Qigong)?	11
Guidelines for Practice	15
Which Qigong	13
A Brief History of Qigong	19
East and West	22
What exactly is "Ch'i or Qi" in the body?	26
Where does Qi come from?	32
How does It work in the body?	36
My Oxygen Theory of Qigong	37
The Meridians and Their Functions	43
The 12 Channels and Flow	44
Hand Positions in Qigong	47
Qi Energy	49
How Should I Go About Learning?	53
Preparing for Qigong	54
Simple Exercises.	60
Bed Time Qigong & Affirmation	61
Energy Boost Qigong	63
Basic Training Methods	67
How Does Qigong Compare With Keep Fit, etc.?	71
Overweight People & Underweight People.	73

Kids and Exercise	76
Pregnancy	78
Be whole	78

Basic Exercise Comparisons — 81

Aerobics (solo & group exercises)	81
Body Building & Weights	82
Core Conditioning	84
Dance related	85
Kick/Box exercise	86
Jogging & Walking	87
Yoga & Stretch	89
Qigong	90
Internal Vs. External Exercises	93
Public and Instructor's Advice	95
Avoiding Injury – Important Advice	97

The Basics of Qigong — 103

The Three Basic Postures	103
Basic Breathing Techniques	105
Beginning	107
The Full Breath	107
The First Qigong Technique	110
Second Technique - Eight Qi Gathering Breaths	111
Third Technique - Expanding the Dantian	115
Fourth Technique - Microcosmic Orbit	120
Moving Qi.	123
Qigong Walking	126

Qigong Street Walking/Cycling   128

Other Qigong Exercises (Sundry Qigong Selection)
Opening The Energy Channels   129

    The Roaming Heavenly Dragon   131
    Lifting The Sky Qigong   133
    Carry The Moon Qigong   135
    Dynamic Qigong   136
    Four Directional Breathing   139

Breathing Exercises for a Purpose   143
    Examples   143
    Meditations   150
    Advanced Qigong   155

Tiandidao Baduanjin: The Eight Strands of Silk Brocade
    Introduction & History   159
    Styles & Comparisons   162
    General Advice   166
    Exercise Check List   171
    The Seated Set   173
    Basic Standing Set   188
    Basic Advanced Set   201
The Role of Baduanjin in Exercise   211
Registered TTT Baduanjin Instructors   215

Personal Notes Space   217
The author's background.   219

Other Books in This Series
    (Practical Taoist Arts)   221

INTRODUCTION

Dear Reader, to make things easier for you pronunciations will be placed in quotes ("speech marks") like the first example in the paragraph below.

Qigong, sometimes written as Ch'i Kung, (is always pronounced like "Chee gong"). It is one of many ancient Chinese health and fitness developments. The Chinese have for thousands of years been probably the greatest inventors on earth. When it comes to looking, learning, understanding and creating, they certainly lead the way. Many other Nations had "great leaders", who rape, pillage and live off the back of other people's toils and China has had its share of those as well, but it really stands out by the fact that it has also had some truly remarkable leaders, not only of men, but of culture too.

Five thousand years ago China had a very civilised culture. Venetian merchant and adventurer Marco Polo, who travelled from Europe to Asia in 1271–95, was greeted in China by an enthusiastic and friendly people. During his trip he had suffered from tiredness and eye strain. A Chinese Official had him see a Doctor right away. He was examined and prescribed eye glasses; unheard of in the West at that time. He was also given Ginseng, to revive his body, given a good diet and shown some simple Qigong to revive his energy. To understand this in perspective you need to know what was happening in England, Italy, France, Spain or even Germany at that time. In regards to developments on par with spectacles, or other Chinese inventions, not a lot. In fact the Britons of that era were living in mud, squalor and most still had huts made of sticks and mud, whilst a few rulers were living in castles and then most did not have glass for their windows, let alone glass for eyes! The Chinese have always been years ahead in invention, yet oddly have never really bothered to do much with it. Qigong was something for the people, not a 'saleable' product, so it was passed on from person to person, family to family, its sole purpose to promote good health.

Take as an example of enterprise the Yellow Emperor, Huang Ti ("Hwang Dee"). He set about understanding Taoism and Taoist practises. With his team of helpers he collated and examined information, facts and figures from far and wide. He wrote books about the resulting findings and was said to be the father of Taoism after then spreading the knowledge back into the public domain. In 'The Yellow Emperor's Canon of Internal Medicine', the earliest known surviving medical work, it said about breathing exercises, "When a person is completely at ease, free of desire and ambition, one will get the genuine energy in order and one's mind concentrated... one must breathe the spiritual energy by concentrating one's mind and relaxing the muscles." This may be the earliest mention of Qigong exercises and was written in the time of his life between 2690-2590 BC. It was a great task that he and his assistants took upon themselves to study, collect and put into print all of the findings on health studies. Some modern scholars seem to think that this great work was actually written in the Han dynasty, making it earlier.

The book in which the philosophical principles are outlined, and it is these principles which are applied to Qigong and the other Arts, dates back to before 2,400 years BC. This is the I-Ching ("Yee Jing") or 'Book of Changes' and discusses all of Nature's variations in a very compact manner. It is recorded that people living in the Shang Dynasty, 1766-1154 BC, used pointed stones to stimulate points on the meridians (channels through which the Qi flows), so obviously quite a bit was known about Qi then.

In recent times Qigong has been in the world news, but mainly for the wrong reasons. Falun Gong was in the news around 2005-6 as the Chinese Communist Government was persecuting them relentlessly, as they have done with any large autonomous organisation. Like many other governments, who live in a constant state of paranoia, they banned any large meetings or popular groups which were not under the control of the government. In this case they banned the meetings of a group of people who met under the Falun Gong banner. Their excuse was that were a few people being 'subversive' (please excuse any apparent cynicism: what, surely not as subversive as the government can be?!), but of course they could not prove this damning claim. Falun Gong was reported to have helped thousands of people to better health. The Communists also shut down many other popular Qigong Health Centres and Hospitals depriving the people of their choice of health care, the popular theory behind this being because they were not state controlled – this being an unfortunate mistake that most major governments seem to make, thinking that "control equals power", but as Lao Tzu said, "A wise ruler sets his people free, therefore they follow him. A Foolish ruler binds his people with chains and rules, therefore they rebel." This has caused an ironic backlash which has brought more traditional Chinese Arts to the West and has helped promote and preserve them and more westerner's health – as they say, "Every cloud has a silver lining"! Now the Chinese people are inheriting smog, junk food, cancer induced by smoking, obesity and traffic jams to go with their new westernised industrial lifestyle.

Research and Development.
In Asia much research has gone into Traditional Medicine, in particular Traditional Chinese Medicine (TCM). Some of the Chinese hospitals and medical institutions are among the finest and most advanced in the world. The Chinese were quick to learn of the dangers of drugs and their wider, deeper background holds the belief that it is unwise to surgically remove parts of the body in the belief that this will cure disease. Their understanding is that the disease does not stem from the infected or affected part, but from other areas; the illness is merely a symptom, not the cause.

Qigong is playing a growing part in modern medicine and in some Chinese Medical Institutions they have conducted clinical experiments with patient's consent and preference using Weiqi instead of anaesthetic drugs; Wei = External or Universal, Qi = Energy or Life Force, hence Weiqi is a method of harnessing and transmitting Universal Qi to a patient, usually through a Medium, a person who is able to do such things. All of the operations were successful, as were operations and cures using acupuncture before them. Patients suffer no pain, no after effects from drugs and in many cases were able to watch the operation and chat to the doctors at the time. Weiqi, like radio waves, can be transmitted from one person to another. I have had personal successes using this method. It can be employed at close quarters or even at a distance, sometimes to a person on the the other side of the world. My Taoist Arts Master, Shih-fu Soo, C. Chee, was the first person I ever saw performing this (1975-9). The fist person to mention this factor in a book for westerners was Shih-fu Wong, Kiew Kit.

Dr. Stephen T. Chang, author of 'The Complete System of Self-Healing Internal Exercises', claims that humans spend most of their lives fulfilling two basic physical needs to maintain, nourish, revitalise and prolong their lives. "These are:
1. Consumption – eating, drinking, etc.
2. Motion
   a. Mind; e.g. thinking, reasoning, etc.
   b. Body; movement and general functions of the body.
   c. Sex."

This logically breaks down existence into basic parts or principles but obviously does not include other human aspects, such as the need for emotional comfort, gratification and other psychological 'needs'. However, he goes on to say that if these basic needs are not fulfilled, and without 'proper' consumption of nutrients, then life will shorten, then premature illness and death follow. Dr. Chang advocates the Taoist system of 'revitalisation', a system of mental and physical movements which we call Qigong. He says, "The Internal exercises heal and energise the internal organs – the keys to youth, immunity against disease and true health". This is where the far older and more highly developed Chinese health system differs from Western health care, thankfully. Nourishing, protecting and maintaining the internal organs is the one most important thing that you can do in your life. In Chinese Medicine there is one thing though which is even more important than the internal organs, the Mind. If the Mind is not kept healthy and in control of one's daily actions, then it may stagnate, become ill and not have the wherewithal to look after the internal organs properly.

In Dr. Chang's list, Mind comes in second place. That is because logically consumption comes first. Without food (nutrition) and oxygen, the mind can not work properly because the brain is 'starved' of life giving essentials. Hence in Taoist Qigong you will find that Diet is the first thing which should be attended to. This logical order extends down the list. If we do not move then circulation in the body slows down and we get eventual stagnation, like a ditch where water does not flow through or has no movement. Movement is essential to life. The exercises of Qigong are not just movement, but 'designer movement', they are designed to move the limbs or body in certain ways so as to exercise internally using external movements, open up energy channels and increase qi, restore balance and enhance health, immunity, digestion, circulation, etc.; the positive effects are almost endless, like ripples extending from a pebble splash in a large pond.

In third place he lists sex. This is because humans have two basic animal functions, to survive and to procreate. Humans are animals and like other animals on this planet humans share many common traits, with one exception, no other animal messes up its environment as badly as humans do! Procreation is the basic need to reproduce, ensuring survival of the species. When most young people reach puberty they seem to have only one thing on their minds, sex. Often, the males are oblivious to the female reasons for looking for a 'mate'. This is because the female of the species is driven more by hormones which drive her to look for a strong, dominant male who will give her good offspring and protect the family. Sadly, in modern society, nine times out of ten this all goes horribly wrong. Since the development of birth control, and various other forms of liberation from responsibility, many humans allow their selves to go out of balance, sexual gratification and its accompanying physical feelings being allowed to come to the forefront, while mental and emotional aspects are held back or disguised, suppressed by emotional fear of involvement, let downs (being emotionally hurt) or other fears. Practising Qigong and understanding the harmonious principles of Tao, many of these problems can be avoided and life can be extended as well as made more pleasant.

One of the body's main energy centres is situated close to the sexual organs. In Qigong, Internal Yoga and other associated Arts, this centre is connected with sex and sexuality. In theory, if sex becomes the most predominant force in one's life, then this centre will be working at full power. Others may not, if the person is not looking after themselves and therefore not 'fully functioning'. Qigong gives balance, enhancing other centres too. The main energy centres in Qigong are described as 'energy gates', sometimes called 'elixir fields' or 'chakras'.

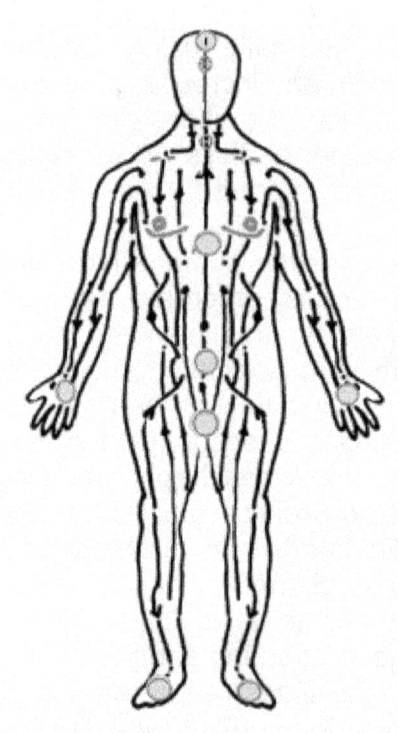

Energy Centres.
In the illustration on the left these 'Primary' centres and 'gates' have been highlighted with grey circles. They are, (1) The Niwangung and Bahui, on top of the head, Pineal and Pituitary Glands. (2) the Huiyin at the Perineum, between the sexual organs and the anus, linked with the sexual glands. (3) the Laogong points on the palms of the hands (P9) and the Yongquan points on the soles of the feet, both called 'wellspring points'. (4) The 'Third-eye' point, between the eyebrows. (5) The heart-level, situated by the Thymus. (6) The Dantian, or Heavenly Elixir, situated in the centreline of the torso and associated with Adrenal and Solar-plexus functions. There is a strong theory and connection with the main glands of the body (The Seven Glands Theory) and in Medical Qigong it is believed that Qigong practice will help the health of these glands and therefore eliminate many health problems; combined with proper nourishment in diet and other senses too, never by itself as all body/mind functions are interlinked. There is another gland associated energy centre at the throat, shown but not listed here. You will also see on the above Illustration that there are points on the feet and hands, these are main energy points but not associated with the glands. They are, Wellspring Point or Yongquan (sole of foot) and P9 on palms of hands.

Heaven and Earth.
The energy centres at the top of the head are linked with Heaven. The centre at the Huiyin point, base of spine, linked with Earth. Between them is the spine, the 'stairway to Heaven', as it is known. As well as concentrating qi at the Lower Dantian, many practitioners raising the qi along the spine to help not only health but enlightenment. The centres are representative of the Great Cosmos, or Universe. The 'centre' of your Universe is the Lower Dantian and the other energy centres and main points represent Universal sub-systems and circuits. Going into details of these serves no purpose in this book, so suffice it to say that one can travel deeper into the realms of Qigong where Energy Channel Theory is linked to Spiritual Qigong practice which is practised for enlightenment, amongst other things. Perhaps the main point to list in the Energy Channel Theory is that the Universe emits many kinds of Qi which vibrate at different frequencies. The Energy Channels and Energy Centres function separately but harmoniously to keep the system working, also using qi. By practising various Forms or methods of Qigong it is possible to "cleanse" these channels or centres, fine tune and then "boost" their performance. This connects Universal Energy with Human functions, body, Mind and Spirit, to elevate one's health, awareness and clarity, etcetera, resulting in what we might simply call "Tuning in with the Universe (Tao)".

The Three Dantian.
Often in Qigong three energy centres are used more than others as a centre of focus. These are, the Lower Dantian (Below the navel), the Middle Dantian (heart level) and the Upper Dantian (between the eyebrows). These centres are ranked by some as being the most important. The Lower Dantian is the central gatherer for Qi and also Distributor and is associated with the vital essence. The Middle Dantian is associated with Fire, ego, emotion and consciousness. The Upper Dantian is associated with wisdom and spirituality. The focus on these three centres in no way detracts from the usefulness and importance of other Qigong methods, just sometimes preferred by those who are trying to aim for enlightenment and spirituality by raising the Qi levels in these important centres along the centre-line.

There are other theories that link Qigong practice to the nervous systems (Nerve Theory), circulation (Circulation Theory) and general functions of the internal organs – as treated in acupressure or acupuncture. I have my own theory (Oxygen Theory) on how Qigong effects the quality of the body tissues and therefore all processes, discussed later on in this book. This knowledge, outlined above, with many medical experiments and claims to health or healing, goes to show what a powerful tool such a simple exercise practice can be.

Qigong Goes West.
In the western hemisphere Qigong is becoming popular for its many health benefits. Many practitioners of Chinese Martial Arts also practice methods of Qigong. Often a student may be lacking in energy, unhealthy or showing symptoms of illness and imbalance. His teacher may then prescribe some Qigong exercises. Through this, an interest sprung up in Qigong as it was realised very quickly what a simple yet powerful tool it was. In my own experience I had discovered the power of Qi (Prana) in Indian Arts, and when I started traditional Taoist Arts with Grandmaster C. Chee Soo, was amazed and impressed by the many formalized and well developed methods that the Chinese had. Shih-fu Soo taught in the UK from as early as the 1950's, but was hardly known by more than a handful then. When I began Teacher Training classes with him in 1975, the secretary gave me a printed extract of a Press article from the Evening Post, Thursday October 7th, 1971. It spanned two pages and detailed how Shih-fu Soo ran a free clinic, the 'Hoimar Brocade' at 377 Edgware Road, London W2. Around those times. He had over 2,000 'patients', as the Press called them, (he called them 'friends') who came to him. Some were friends to begin with, others recommended by their friends, or by Chee Soo's students. There were many people who had been through the hospital system, from virtually one end of the chain to the other, all without expectation of relief and often being told by hospital doctors that there was no hope for them, they were "incurable". It had got to a point where even NHS Specialists were throwing up their hands and saying, "Sorry, I can do no more. If you want, why don't you go see that Chinese man who runs a free clinic in London?"

Mrs Janet Slow from Northampton was one visitor to the centre. She had "Multiple Sclerosis" for 23 years, according to the report. She told the Press, "Four years ago it was so bad I could hardly put one leg in front of the other and after a heart attack my hands were severely afflicted. I couldn't go to work, although I did hairdressing at home, partly as therapy for my hands. Then I came to Cliff, I lost two Stones [in weight], which I'm really delighted about, and for the first time I can go out to work. Now I'm a Ward Orderly in a Northampton hospital, I enjoy it and I see a lot of people who are much worse off than me. I'm tired but I feel well – I've so much more energy, I can run upstairs. The Multiple Sclerosis Association considers me the Wonder Girl!"

Of course, Qigong was not the only thing that helps, but also your general lifestyle and diet. The Taoist Long Life Diet, (See: 'Tai Chi Diet' - ISBN: 9780954293284), is the most wonderful and natural 'food sense' in the world. Qigong, the most wonderful energy training and health giving exercise and Taoist Kung Fu... just wonderful!

In writing this book it is my hope to enlighten the reader who has never done any training in this simple yet life transforming method and to encourage you to go out, find a really good teacher and practice every day. Hopefully, in the process of reading this, a few myths will be dispelled as well as answering a few unanswered questions, revealing a few 'secrets' and piece together parts of a mysterious puzzle which has intrigued many people for hundreds of years: "Is that all?" I hear a few people say in jest. Yes, sorry, lack of ambition, that's my problem! ;-) Oh look, the first 'Emoticon' in a book?! What about that Oxford? :-P

My hope is that this little book helps in some way to change the attitudes of people around the world, especially in the western hemisphere, thus changing society for the better and getting rid of some of the modern worthless and destructive cultural 'hiccups' like drugs (including herbal highs and caffeine drinks) and smoking. Enjoy something natural. Enjoy Qigong.

WHAT IS CH'I KUNG (QIGONG)?

Qigong (Trad. Chinese. 氣功) or Energy Training is a practical scientific Art of exercise which uses both the mind and body to harness the natural energies of the Universe and Earth. It is a range of simple exercises with many variations that are designed to improve the body's bioenergy and metabolic functions, therefore improving health overall. This reformation takes place from the inside, working outwards throughout the body. Qigong can also have a profound effect upon the spiritual essence of the human and with regular practice can help a person to transcend from the base to the higher levels of consciousness and living to better and clearer plains of power and perception.

More generally speaking it is a form of Chinese exercise which was mainly developed by those people who are known as Taoists ("Dowists"). To many this name conjures up religious connections and it would be true to say that there are some Taoists who would call it a religion, but this is not true. Virtually any belief or form of actions can be labelled a 'religion', but in Taoism ("Daoism") the true aim is not to blindly follow but to free oneself from earthly shackles and become harmonised with Nature, Universal Nature, TAO ("Dow"). Many people's actions and philosophies have in the past been misinterpreted by those seeking to bathe in the wake of success. If you think about it, Christ was not a Christian, he was a Jew. He was an exceptional man and followed a set of ways and values which produced his particular healing and counselling skills. To the Jews of that era everyone was 'like unto God' and all life was special. It was only his later followers that coined the phrase Christian. Likewise, Siddārtha Gautama or Lord Buddha was not a Buddhist, nor did he found Buddhism, his followers followed him and called it Buddhism (Buddha means 'Enlightened One', he was dubbed Lord as he was the son of a warrior caste Prince, like a Lord). The Taoists follow Tao, which means 'Way', or Nature's Way: life, the universe and everything. Nature has no religious ways but is purely the Form of creation, living, action and inaction within life and the

Universe as we know it. There is no one founder and no one accredited creator or leader in Taoism, although much of the study and development have been accredited to Emperor Huang Ti and the great philosopher Lao Tzu - ancients who dedicated most of their life to understanding Tao. Quite simply, the object of Taoism is not to follow blindly, or be a hanger-on, but to study, practice and develop one's self in order to improve the quality of life and reach one's own personal enlightenment. Then, hopefully, pass it on to a few others. Thus the world can gradually be improved. Taoists have for centuries studied, experimented and developed methods of living a longer, better and healthier life. In the process many forms of Qigong have been created.

One of the earliest mentions of Qigong was in a diary type record written by a Taoist called Xunxun, the 'Jing Ming Religious Record', this was in the Qin (Ch'in) Dynasty (c.221-c.206 B.C and called the 'Elaboration of Qi Gong', but no explanation of the term was given. Later, in 1935, Donghao wrote 'Special Therapy for Tuberculosis', which was published by the Zhonghua Press. However, it was not until much later in 1953 that the author Liu Guizheng wrote 'Practice on Qigong Therapy' that the name was explained and accepted as a recognised title. This was then rapidly accepted by other schools as a formal title for the Arts. In his book, Liu says, "Qi means respiration, while Gong means continuous regulation of breathing in different postures." As you will come to see later on in this book, there is far more to Qigong than meets the eye, that is, far more than just breathing and posturing.

Qigong derives from two basic Chinese characters, Ch'i = Essence or Energy, can also imply 'energy taken from breath'. Kung (pronounced "Gong" or "Gung"), means to acquire through labours, but can also imply 'to regulate or control'. Hence Qigong is generally taken as a simplified title to mean 'Energy Training' and implies the use of concentration and willpower to attain the skills and the desired results: like a great Artist who can take years to acquire the right techniques and temperament. So whilst Qigong is fundamentally simple, to reach its highest levels can take many years.

Which Qigong?

There are many forms or versions of Qigong, including the popular Taoist, Buddhist and Confucian exercises, influenced by their respective philosophies, then there are the Medical Qigong exercises, used as specialised exercises, and finally the Martial Qigong, used to develop strength and 'Inner Power'. Many cross-over into the territory of the other. For example, Baduanjin (Pa T'uan Chin), which has general health values, both internal and external, plus medical and martial values too. Let us take a look at the main fields of Qigong practice:

Qigong in Health.

A wide field which covers anything from health improvements to health rebalancing or self-healing. This practice may take the form of the sitting, standing or laying down postures, depending on ability. Concentration may be on Dantian or Abdominal Breathing, a set of defined movements, such as Baduanjin, or something more specific for rebuilding one's health after illness or accident. As a preventative medicine or therapy Qigong really finds its niche. By performing some sort of Qigong routine every day it is possible that you will ward off many kinds of illnesses, reduce stress, reduce risk of cancer, improve circulation, help eliminate toxins, improve tissue quality (internal and external), clear the mind, raise energy levels, alleviate arthritis and much more.

Qigong Therapy.

This is a term used to describe the application of Qi to cure or strengthen another person. Exercises may be taught by a Doctor, Therapist or a Qigong Instructor. Baduanjin is often classified as Qigong Therapy or Self-healing Qigong. There are three basic methods in the Qigong Therapy application:
1. To transmit one's qi to a "patient" with the intention of healing or redressing the balance of a Meridian, function, etcetera.
2. To rebalance a person's or your own Qi by the guided use of herbs, acupressure / acupuncture, etcetera.
3. To recommend specific exercises for a purpose.

Any one, two or all three of the above methods may be used according to need and the depth of the problem.

Martial Qigong.
This can take the form of specific exercises to improve power, strengthen parts of the anatomy, increase energy focus or expression, but more often than not will include 'every day' qigong exercises, such as Baduanjin. It can also be used in self-healing where injuries have occurred in fighting practice. Martial Qigong is a specialised field and can not be attempted by untrained individuals as self-damage could easily occur; just like within any practise, sport or occupation, except malpractice in Qigong can cause serious imbalances that can lead to serious health problems; think of it as being akin to practising surgery on yourself without training!

Two Basic Methods.
Qigong is done in two basic methods, stationary (Yin) or moving (Yang), with many variations. In both methods the emphasis is placed on correct breathing formulas and proper mental concentration. In Yin Qigong one may be lying down, seated on a basic chair, seated in a meditation posture or standing up in one of several poses. In Yang Qigong the movement is dictated by the need and desired outcome. Everyone must start with the foundational methods in all skills, here it is correct breathing technique. There are no short cuts in Qigong.

Stationary Qigong.
In this method the body is still, yet inside there is great movement and concentration. The Mind focusses internally and the Qi is moved, centred at specific points or used to "wash" the energy channels. Qi can also be transmitted from one person to another whilst static.

Moving Qigong.
In moving Qigong it is the movements of the outer body which help induce specific effects that take place from the inside. The Mind still guides and controls or regulates the Qi, but the postures are also important as correct posture strengthens effect; this is especially so in general Medical Qigong and Martial Qigong. There are some general guidelines to practising Qigong, these should be studied and followed.

To find the right type of Qigong training for you, you should first and always find a suitably qualified instructor or medical practitioner who is familiar with the above aspects. This is not to say that you could join a good class of general Qigong, like Baduanjin, for example.

Health Qigong is practised by anyone wishing to improve their own health. This has many beneficial effects, including the improvement of overall body tissue, blood, brain and bio-functions, to giving more energy and better healing power. Exercises need to be shown and explained personally by a very experienced practitioner, then monitored.

Medical Qigong is usually administered or taught by an experienced health practitioner for specifically diagnosed imbalances or health problems. Medical Qigong should not be taught as part of a general public qigong class, unless they are TCM students, as it could have undesired effects on a otherwise "healthy" system.

Martial Qigong is again something which should only be taught by a high-level practitioner, and then only to select students. An example of bad practice: In 2007 a colleague told me of a demonstration by a Chinese teacher in Sydney, Australia, the man threw a Qi Punch out into the audience at an apparently targeted westerner. He later saw the westerner as he was getting changed and saw he had a massive bruise coming out on his chest and was visibly shaken, but afraid to say anything. This could have dire consequences on his health and could even kill him; not least by blood clotting! As far as I am concerned, any teacher of Taijiquan or Taoist Kung Fu who does that kind of trick does not deserve to be called Shih-fu.

Guidelines for Practice.
As with all disciplines, there are guidelines which have been set out by the experts and based upon years of study. It is important that these are understood. Many Westerners dabble in Qigong, thinking that just because something is written in a book that they can emulate the postures and basic advice to achieve the same kinds of results as the author. This is not possible, you need instruction, personal instruction and good

instruction. The advice below represents just some of the advice which, in time, is what you may receive from an instructor; sometimes this may come only after asking questions, given the busy nature of a group session.

- Fixed Ideas and Time. A regular schedule is required for practice, but do not be alarmed or upset if you have to break the routine. Just be firm that you will come back to it and make time for it later. Sometimes you may see a "window" of opportunity to grab some extra practice, like when walking the dog in the countryside, so take it, such opportunity can be rare these days.
- Goal setting. In one word, "Don't!". Although you should have regular practice you can not set goals beyond that. For example, feeling the Qi rise up the spine, or feeling that warm sensation in the hands or at the Dantian. These things will happen when they happen. If you are looking for them then you will not be training properly and will also miss the point of the exercise. Remember, Qi is guided by the Mind, so if you are thinking about feeling a tingling sensation in your right hand, then that is where your Qi will be. If you were meant to be concentrating on the Dantian, then you will have spoiled the exercise and therefore will not achieve the correct results. Do only what you are supposed to be doing and concentrate only on the guidelines for that specific exercise. Progress will come and when you do feel sensations just acknowledge them and then continue as normal.
- Speed and Short cuts. Neither is applicable to Qigong. Trying to speed up results or take short cuts may only result in frustration and despair, then failure. Be prepared to develop patience, concentration and endurance. Qigong takes time, a long time, it is a distant goal which is worth reaching, so take your journey at a steady pace with this in mind.
- Shock and Change. If we receive a mental shock (trauma), such as the loss of a loved one, then the Mind and the body (governed to a degree by the Mind) will need time to readjust and settle. Likewise, if your environment suddenly changes, like moving from a

warm climate to a cold climate, or visa-versa, then again time is needed for natural readjustment. Do not practice your Qigong if you are deeply disturbed or unsettled. Rest, seek calm before continuing.

- Personal Environment. Just as it is important not to practice in dusty or dirty places it is also important to note personal hygiene. Wearing dirty clothes, feeling sweaty or itchy is not conducive to good practice. Always make sure that you feel comfortable. If you are sweaty or wet, stay out of the wind, especially if you are relaxed as when you sweat your skin pores open and this could leave you prone to Cold or other ailments. Being too warm or too cold is something else to avoid.
- Distractions. There will no doubt be times when distractions come. You may hear a telephone ringing, someone at the door or somebody calling you. There may also be times when you feel insects biting you, birds flapping nearby, bees or wasps hovering around your head. Any sudden distraction will take your mind away from practice. Under such circumstances remain calm – bring your mind back to the Dantian – take some deep but controlled breaths and centre your qi at the Dantian. One of the things which happens in qigong is a sudden itching or tingling sensation somewhere on the body. At first this may seem strange and distracting, learn to ignore it and it will pass; this is only the natural process of Qi as it adjusts, heals or redistributes itself around the system. Sometimes you will feel one of your 'acupoints' being adjusted, for example.
- Clothing. Tight clothing, including tight belts or waist bands, women's Bra's, corsets, etc., will reduce circulation and restrict natural movement. Wear loose, comfortable clothing and (as suggested elsewhere in this book) cotton is best as man made fibres like nylon can cause the Qi to be dispersed or misguided.
- Sexual Activity. As mentioned elsewhere, being celibate for six months to a year is of use when training. It is also inadvisable to have sex within a 24 hour period before or after specialised Qigong practice. This traditionally is extended to all Qigong, but more especially Martial Qigong or Therapy (Medical) Qigong. In TCM theory

sperm is transmuted to Qi. As sperm is made up of a very high amount of proteins, there may be a dietary link to this theory, but nevertheless depletion of the sperm can lead to a breakdown of transformation of the body's healing and building processes after Qigong if ejaculation has occurred. Women also benefit from celibacy as this can save energy and if you think about the huge amounts of energy required by the female's body to heal and repair, especially after monthly Periods, this makes sense in that context alone. For those in an active relationship the balancing of the energy centres and correct diet are very important.

Other details could be added to this list but the essential points are there. It is worthwhile studying these guidelines and contemplating them for a while before beginning your Qigong practice. Much advice is, or should be, common sense, such as not exercising just after meals, etcetera.

See Also:
Advice in the Baduanjin section (p.160-164). Rather than making one huge section on advice, which may put readers off by its length and depth, it seemed more prudent to split items up and even repeat some important key points. Everyone should read this, especially instructors.

Summary.
Overall you can see that Qigong is something to be taken seriously, it is not something which can be dabbled with or taken frivolously. Yes, it most certainly is possible to try some Qigong, just on a curiosity basis, to see if you like it; all Instructors should know some simple exercise which allows a person to sample Qigong without changing anything that can not be undone. Qigong is not like going for a walk, going to the Gym or taking part in a Sport, it is a serious Art which should be undertaken with a mind to making a life time of practice and improvement. Always understand what it is that you are taking on, then take and heed advice from a knowledgeable instructor.

A BRIEF HISTORY OF QIGONG

The fist knowledge of Qigong ("Chee Gong") was from some copper ware items found in China dating from the Shang Dynasty (c. 1600 BC - c. 1046 BC)) and early Zhou Dynasty (Wade-Giles Translation: Chou Ch'ao; 1122 BC to 256 BC). These showed images of ancient Chinese people doing exercises for health which researchers believe is Qigong.

In 'The Yellow Emperor's Canon of Internal Medicine', the earliest known surviving medical work, it said about breathing exercises, "When a person is completely at ease, free of desire and ambition, one will get the genuine energy in order and one's mind concentrated..... One must breathe the spiritual energy by concentrating one's mind and relaxing the muscles." This may be the earliest mention of Qigong exercises and was written in the time of his life between 2690-2590 BC. The Yellow Emperor was known as Huang Ti ("Hwang Di"), it was a great task that he and his assistants studied, collated and put into print all of the findings on health studies. Some modern scholars seem to think that this great work was actually written in the Han dynasty, making it earlier.

The book in which the philosophical principles are outlined, which may applied to Qigong and the other Arts, dates back to before 2,400 years BC. This is the I-Ching ("Yee Jing") or 'Book of Changes'. It is recorded that people living in the Shang Dynasty, 1766-1154 BC, used pointed stones to stimulate points on the meridians (channels through which the Qi flows), so obviously quite a bit was known about Qi then.

Famous Taoist philosopher Lao Tzu, real name Li Ehr, wrote of Qigong and 'breath of life' in his poem on the 'Way of Nature' the Tao Te Ching ("Dow De Jing"). This awesome work was written in the sixth century BC. A good translation is recommended reading and there is happily a wonderful translation available by Witter Bynner, the late American poet, 'The Way of Life – according to Lao Tzu', search for this on the Internet.

Taoist: Chen Tuan (陳摶)
a.k.a. Chen Po (871-989)

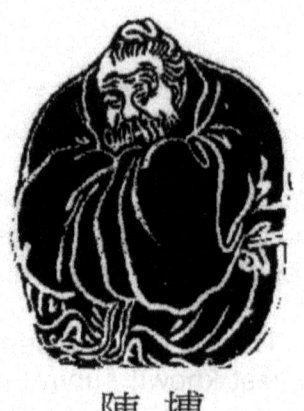

陳摶

Chen Tuan (Given Sage name 'Chen Xi Yi') was a legendary Taoist sage and son of China. According to some Taoist schools, who like to claim him as a founder, he lived a solitary life in the 'Nine Room Cave' on Mount Wu Tang ("Wudang") – one of the many caves carved out of the vast Wudang complex. The picture above right, taken from an ancient wood-block, depicts him sitting in his cave, huddled in his robes. He grew up in a village called Ching Yun and reputedly spent lots of time in his youth playing on the shore where he was particularly fascinated by the flow and fluidity of water; In Taoist Philosophy Water is not only the most subtle element but also the strongest.

Later in his life, while at Mount Hua, one of the five sacred Wudang or 'Five Peaks' mountains of China, he is said to have created the Kung Fu system Liu He Ba Fa (Six Harmonies and Eight Methods), often called 'Water Form Boxing' as his fascination of water influenced his styling. Alongside this well known Internal Martial Art, he is also said to be associated with a method of chi (energy) cultivation known today as Taiji Ruler, Sleeping Meditation 'Erh Shih Ssu Shih Tao Yin Fa' or 24 methods of directing Qi – 24 seated and standing exercises that are designed to prevent diseases or pathogens that occur during seasonal change. Altogether he had a very productive life full of truly great achievements.

The popular story says that Chen Tuan had planned a career at the Imperial court, but failed the state examination and became a hermit sage and travelled instead. He was also said to be conversant with the Confucian classics, history, and the theories of various schools of thought. In his legends he was said to be fond of Buddhist philosophy, medical principles, astronomy and geography, and famous for his poems as well.

Chen Tuan liked to study the I Ching ("Yee Jing") - Book of Changes - , which according to colleagues, he was reputedly unable to put down.

There have been many exercises, or sets, accredited to many people. Among these are Jingong, Daoyin, Tuna, Xingqi, Neiyanggong, Yangshenggong and many more. All of these have different and sometimes exotic names, but in essence they share similar functions. In several books, published around the 1930's, two main characters were used in describing these exercises, 'Qi Gong', although no explanation was apparently made for this at the time. Later this became a generic name for any exercise using breathing and mind control of energy in its goal. As mentioned earlier, Qigong loosely means 'energy training' but can also be translated in accordance with the functions of the exercises, such as using the mind to direct, lead or control the flow of Qi, a common feature of many of these exercises.

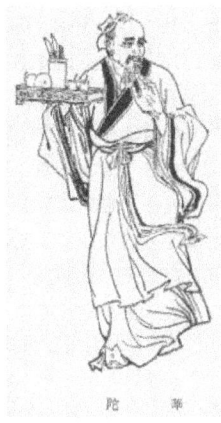

One famous and popular system of Qigong exercise called Wuqinxi (Wu Chin Hsi), 'Five Animal Play', is accredited to Doctor Hua To[1], (? - to – 208 AD) the famous physician, he developed this set of Qigong exercises around the third century BC. These exercises mimicked the movements of the tiger, monkey, deer, bear and bird to generate healing Qi and strength. The theory behind this was that all these creatures relied upon natural movements for their health and strength, so mimicking these movements may help humans to be as strong or nimble as them.

Much later, after many, many other doctors and scholars had produced refined methods of Qigong, a man called Da Mo, who was a Buddhist teacher, stayed at the Shaolin Temple in

---

[1] Who do you think performed the first Heart Transplant and when? Dr Christian Barnard in the UK in the 1960's? Wrong. The first ever transplant was performed by Dr. Hua To nearly three hundred years before Christ was born; he used bamboo acupuncture needles and performed it with success on twin brothers who volunteered!

Son Shan Mountain region of Honan. He eventually spent nine years in seclusion there and developed another set of "animal play" exercises, the 'I Chin Ching' ("Yee Jin Jing"), or 'Muscle Change Method'. These were designed originally to strengthen the muscles, ligaments and tendons of the Shaolin Monks who suffered many injuries during hard Martial Arts training; probably because they spent much time sitting around learning Buddhist scriptures at that time. The movements of I Chin Ching are hard and demand much strength, much more so than Pa Tuan Chin, for example, but within the hardness is softness and the mind must be composed with harmonious breathing. This is often called "Hard Qigong", meaning external rather than internal, often resembling dynamic tension exercises.

So the developments went on and still do. Now Qigong has spread from China and is taking on a world-wide role as a famed healing and refreshing method. In these days when stress produces more illness than most other negative health factors there are many more people learning the traditional exercises and teaching in just about every town and city. There are many Chinese Arts instructors or Shih-fu ("Shifu" or "Shir-fu", said abruptly) like myself who are attempting to develop the Arts further. In my own case I like to cross-reference against western Orthodox medical information where possible - not that Orthodox Medicine knows much at all in the field of Energy, as it is traditionally based on strong drugs and surgery - common effects and symptoms are easier to cross-reference.

East and West.

Qigong has been extensively developed in China. However, in the west many people have still not heard of it. In the 1960's I studied meditation and yoga, and found some very unusual side-effects – these I now know to be Qi. In 1975, even though an 'outsider', I was invited to train in the Teacher's Training classes of one Professor Clifford Chee Soo. He taught Taoist Arts, including Feng Sou ("Fung Shaow") Kung Fu, Li or Lee Family Style Taijiquan, Taoist Yoga, Qigong, Taoist 'Long Life' Diet and healing. Attending his classes was amazing as his Qi was strong and he could project it from himself to someone else too, with considerable ease. I have many memorable stories from those days, and not all my own either as most of his other student-teachers had plenty of eye-witnessed events to talk about too. Shih-fu Soo's knowledge of Qi and his ability to transmit it were like nothing I had ever seen or heard of before, or since!

One of the things which struck me during a session when we were learning another new series of Taoist Yoga exercises. Lao Bah mentioned that what we were doing was part of a series known as Eight Strands of Brocade. Why this struck me was because I had already come across a series of exercises called Eight Strands of Silk Brocade and they were nothing like these ones. This spurred me on to find out as much as possible about the Eight Strands of Brocade (Baduanjin, or Pa Tuan Chin) and its many variations. Some of these variations were, at first sight, average, others alright and a few downright dangerous looking – in terms of medical safety. It was difficult to get reliable information in the 1970's, and not always easy in the 1980's. Through all this I managed to get enough information from around the world to enable me to look at the differing sets and to be able to distinguish between one and another. With my training and background it was possible to look at each exercise in turn for its merits. First of all came practicability. Some variations were clearly unsuitable for someone with a healthy spine, let alone someone who had back problems. There had been a set of Baduanjin developed in Beijing, by a government commissioned Professor, to suit the common people after a realisation for the need of standardisation. However, this was only a basic set and did not include seated for disabled and convalescing, or a more advanced set. Further study and trials ensued. In the late 1980's I introduced Baduanjin as a prelude to learning Taijiquan. This worked very well and the results were remarkable.

In the late 1990's the revised Form was introduced to the UK with complete and revised safer Sets (one seated, two standing) which is now known world-wide as the 'New (Safer) Standardised Set of Baduanjin' (sometimes written in Traditional as Pa T'uan Chin). This Set and method is now being taught and is spreading throughout the UK and Ireland due to some National training courses held in the lovely old city of Cambridge, England. On one of these occasions I recall walking into the long training hall and, as I neared the group of trainees, walking into a huge energy ball of qi around them!

Student-Instructors report many successes from personal use and therapeutic workshops, or regular classes. One of the most common comments being, "It has completely transformed my Qigong practices". The main comment or observation outside of Instructor's personal use is the effect on class members, comments like "They come in looking weary and down, but they leave looking energised and with a big smile on their face!"

The fully inclusive list of the key players or developers would run into thousands, if not hundreds of thousands, many of who's praises have never been sung. In China, mainland and offshore, over the past few decades much research has gone into Traditional Medicine, in particular Traditional Chinese Medicine (TCM). Independent research has also been carried out outside of mainland China, some in Taiwan (Republic of China), UK, USA, Hawaii, Korea and a few other places. Many biologists and physicists have been, and some still are, quite sceptical of claims about Qi being an undetectable (by human eye) force which pervades the body, and world in general. Claims made by Chinese Doctors and Qigong Masters have been ridiculed and many ignorant western medical people regard them as pseudo-scientific. In Taiwan, around 1980, some American and Chinese medical scientists conducted a series of tests and experiments to discover what Qi is and whether it really flows around the energy channels, as stated by acupuncturists. This was done with the co-operation of a respected Acupuncturist and a Qigong Master, as well as the team of scientists from both countries (see next Chapter).

Many students and teachers of Qigong can see Qi leaving the tips of their fingers whilst practising qigong exercises, some can see it in the form of auras around the body. Sometimes, and only with senior students, the effects of Qi are demonstrated and can be felt by them; without first explaining what will happen so they do not know what to expect. Usually this works and the student, without seeing the Master performing, can verify the effects. This form of demonstration is not uncommon in a class situation and is very useful and educational, both for the students and the teachers.

As said above, both in China and outside, studies have or are being conducted between medical scientists and Qigong practitioners to find out more about what Qi is and the effects it has on the body. An extract of one example of a more recent study may be seen below.

Study of microwave radiation component of External Qi of Qigong. By Chuanlian Yao; Jiaqi Shen.

Microwave Conference Proceedings, 1997. APMC apos;97., 1997 Asia-Pacific. Volume 1, Issue , 2-5 Dec 1997 Page(s):57 - 60 vol.1 - Digital Object Identifier 10.1109/APMC.1997.659304

Summary:
The physics of External Qi of Qigong was studied using the microwave radiation component with a 3cm wavelength spectra microwave radiation instrument. Fourteen (14) Qigong masters were invited to join the experiment. External Qi was emitted from the Lau Gong point of the palm (P.9) which was placed 2 cm away from the horn antenna of the microwave radiometer. The paper describes a detection method for External Qi by using X-band microwave radiometry, instrument structure and experimental results.

You can find reference to this experiment on the Internet by typing into a Browser's Search Bar the information in the title. It is too lengthy to include here. There are other experiments and results to be found, not all easy to track down though, so only those truly interested in research will pursue this line of enquiry.

What exactly is Ch'i or Qi in the body?

As I write this I can virtually hear many readers' minds ticking over at high revolutions, saying, "Hang on, so what is Qi then? Are we talking radio waves here?" Yes, and no. I came across a report in the 1980's which gave descriptions of results emanating from the R.o. China and a large modern medical institute there. In the combined experiments conducted between Chinese and American Medical Scientists, involving Medical Doctors, a high-level Acupuncturist and a Qigong Master, the tests conclusively proved that Qi existed. They confirmed, by tracking with sensitive instruments, the 12 Major Meridians and the sub-meridians, all the acupoints and more. They developed a small device, based on an Ampere Meter design, which was sensitive enough to measure the body's bioenergies and then set out to discover exactly what Qi is. Since then I have been passing on this information to my students and have developed a simple exercise to perform in which they can recognise and feel these basic Qi energies.

In mainland China a goal was set to discover what Qi is, the deadline for this was 1977. The experiment was carried out at the Shanghai Traditional Chinese Medicine College with the co-operation of the Shanghai Atomic Nuclear Research Institute and a Qigong Master (not named). The scientists measured Weiqi (External Energy) omitted by the Qigong Master using modern instruments. Again the results pinpointed Infra-red, Static Electricity and Magnetic energies. In conclusion they could say what Qi was, at least partially, but were not sure if these energies were part of the 'carrier' or the actual essence. Fluid changes in the body of the Qigong Master were also noted.

This led the way to a further and much larger experiment which involved even more professional bodies. The Chinese Academy of Science, The National Physical Culture and Sports Commission joined forces with the National Science Commission and the Ministry of Public Health to conduct a more definitive test. They met at the Xi Yuan Guest House in Beijing in July 1978. Qi was again proven beyond doubt that it was a "material" substance. In the Infra-red test, a HD-1 Infra-red Thermometer was used (8-14 micrometer window) to measure the energy omitted by Qigong Master Lin, Hou-sheng. The instrument was placed one metre away from Master Lin's hand as he omitted Qi from his hand Laogong point. Low frequency Infra-red signals were picked up and it was noted that these fluctuated greatly. The signals were compared to those of non-Qigong practitioners and found to be very different and highly pronounced.

In the test for Static, a scientific instrument was placed 2 Cm away from the emission point (Yintang) of Qigong Master Cheng, Zhi-jiu. Master Liu, Jin-rong was measured from 5 Cm away from his emission (Bahui) point. Static charges were measured of between 10-14 – 10-11 Coulomb (an electrical measure named after Charles Augustin de Coulomb and equal to around 100,000 to 1,000,000 Electrons) were recorded and it was also found that these emissions varied when they changed their qigong methods.

The test for magnetic energy was even more remarkable. Master Liu Jin-rong raised his Qi up to his Bahui point (top of the head) whilst another man repeatedly struck the top of his head with a Steel bar; measuring 76 cm in length, 5 cm wide and 4 cm thick. The steel bent with each strike, but Master Liu was completely unhurt. The magnetic detector received strong signals from Master Liu's Bahui point.

A further test using a Niobium-lithium-aluminium Piezoelectric Ceramic Detector, was used to verify Qi omitted by Qigong Master Zhao Wei-fa. His Qi moved the suspended thread and pushed falling ceramic powder dust over one metre forwards! The results were compared to a small electric fan and it was found throughout the experiments that the effect of Qi was entirely different to that of the effects of airflow. This time the Qi was designated as a 'pulse' with a vibration of 50 to 150 Milliseconds, 0.3 Hertz at intervals of 2-20 seconds. The full details are not readily available, but it was recorded that the pulses travelled at a speed of 20-60 centimetres per second over a distance of up to 3 Metres in front of Master Zhao.

Russian Scientists at The Research Institute of Acoustics also carried out an experiment using unconventional X-Ray equipment that can "see" subsonic signals that the human eye can not. Their tests showed a brilliant Aura around the Qigong Master's body and a bright ring of light just above his head. They also experimented with emotions to see what effect this had on the energies. They found that with the emotions of love and excitement the aura became almost "like a firework display" with many colours and stems. Kirlean photography has long since proved that the energy fields around a Qigong Master's fingers are much larger and stronger than those of a non-practitioner. The results of similar pictures can often be seen at Health and Well-being Fairs, recently found in the UK and USA.

A must read book is one by Daniel Reid who has spent much time in R.o. China learning from Lo Teh-Hsiu and other notables. In his book, which I ashamedly still have not had time to read fully but nevertheless appreciate very much as a reference, ' A Complete Guide To Chi-Kung' (ISBN: 1-57062-543-3), he explains some information related to Piezoelectric and energy functions within the realms of Qigong; it is therefore not necessary for me to repeat what others have already said and his book will add to your knowledge and understanding of this deep subject. Go buy it.

While I am not entirely sure what all the energies do or what their functions are within the body, my theory or "educated guess" is that the Low Frequency Modulation Infra-red Microwaves are involved in healing and repair or strengthening the body. What appears to be a form of Static Electrical energy can be used in self-defence, as can Electromagnetic Pulses, which may have a desired affect on someone else's energy field, sending them off-balance or other effects; as dictated by the sender or "transmitter". These two energies also have normal functions within the body, within and governed by the energy channels. The 'static' in the body probably functions within the nervous system and brain. More scientific study is required in this area as the information I require is not available to me right now. The study of Qi is something really quite exciting and largely undiscovered, perhaps in my next life I shall dedicate to that? There you have it, many years study of Qi captured in one measly paragraph!

Here and now I can tell you that the three basic energies or types of Qi in the human body are:
1. Static Electricity (a form of, or with like effects)
2. Low Frequency Modulation Infra-red Microwaves
3. Electromagnetic energy.

It is also possible that Ionic energy and Plasma also play a part in what we call "Qi". It has given me great pleasure to develop a simple exercise which enables someone to feel their Qi, all three basic energies. The looks on people's faces when they feel the electromagnetic energy field is something I always cherish, as well as making me smile – they look like they have just discovered a precious jewel in the desert, and indeed they have found a real gem in the desert of life.

Many Chinese people prefer to practice their Qigong by a waterfall or moving stream as well as under healthy trees. It is said that moving water creates good Qi. Modern day science dealing with energies has partly revealed the reasons why this happens, Ions. Ions are atoms or molecules which have either lost or gained one or more electrons. This gives the Ion a negative or positive charge. Negatively charged Ions have more electrons than protons and is called an Anion (from the Greek 'up'). There are many other sub-categories and many more types of Ion with elemental differences. Without going too deeply into scientific 'technobabble'. Negative Ions are good for your health and moving water is said to release negative ions. These can float in the air near to their creative source. However, negative ions are absorbed by concrete and machinery which then release positive ions. Positive Ions are not good for your health.

Once, when between classes at a city leisure centre which had clothes washing facilities, I conducted my own small experiment. As the washing machines used gallons of water every day, had drains beneath the masses of concrete (moving water), plus water mains pipes of course, this seemed the ideal place to test the Ion theory. If Negative Ions are absorbed through the floors and positive ions are released back out, then in my simple theory there must be lots of negative charge left below the floor in this area. Taking note of my feelings, it seemed as if the surroundings could easily make me tired or drowsy. Sitting on a small wooden bench I began 'heel breathing' exercises as my intent was focussed on drawing negative ions and good Qi up through the floor. It worked! Within five minutes I felt as though I had been plugged in to Blackpool Illuminations. The energy was very strong, easy to feel and had an almost immediate 'lifting' effect.

Ions are present throughout the Universe. The Geophysical Institute of the University of Alaska published a paper after studying and measuring Ion activity. According to them there are approximately 1,000 negative and positive ions per cubic centimetre of outdoor air. These are created by cosmic rays. There are higher concentrations at higher altitudes, like mountain tops (Wudang ;-) and by the sea or waterfalls. The presence is lowered in densely populated city areas, for example. Scientists say that well-being can be improved by using an artificial ion generator, or Ioniser., though they say that they do not know the reason for this. It is interesting to note that Asus, the computer and component manufacturer, has now started building Ionisers into their Laptop machines. Taoists simply *accept* that Qi is good for you as it helps the biological processes. Ionisers are being used in some Asian hospitals in ways that may help in reducing the number of airborne infections. Ionisers used in air purifiers though are said not to work in helping reduce particles, such as dust. If I was considering the purchase of an indoor Ioniser, I would want to do a lot of research first.

Plasma is another substance or matter which has links with Ions. There are many links between various types of energy or matter, perhaps many more will be discovered scientifically in the future. Rumour has it that at the notorious mystery base near Roswell (USA) there has been significant development in Plasma technology resulting in the development of the nicknamed 'Aurora', a plasma powered 'UFO' which can fly at speeds around 8,000 miles per hour, leaving only a small exhaust trace visible only from satellites. The plasma drive harnesses power from Universal energy, Weiqi, as the Taoists call it; the Taoists have been harnessing Weiqi for centuries, but not to fly! In the future deep space travel will be possible using such a source of constant and renewable energy, to use a catch phrase. Then man, with his "head in the heavens", will discover other planets, other life forms and perhaps some startling information; maybe startling to scientists but perhaps not so surprising to Taoists who have believed in the powers of these unseen energies for centuries. These energies are produced by the Universe and support it in many ways. There is much to learn and many connections to make, as far as science goes. Perhaps Taoists, or Life Scientists, have the right idea, live, gain, use these forces and discover more along the way, passing on that information to others in turn.

In my profession it is a task of life, my life, to study, detect, try to understand, dissect and rebuild information relating to the Taoist Arts. Like any life science, the payment for this is satisfaction. This is what many thousands of Taoists have been doing since Taoism was first discovered. In the field of Qigong, I declare that at first, and like many people, I was confused or bewildered by the concepts and practices of qigong. After many years of study and development though it becomes quite clear, and simple. We are Tao.

There have been some experiments which have accidentally discovered aspects of Qi in the western hemisphere in the past, but ignored. One was the 'electric wind' experiment. If my memory serves me well enough, this was discovered by a French scientist, probably around the early 1600's. He discovered that if you held a pin or needle between the tips of your finger and thumb, then made the point of it approach a candle flame, the candle flame would start to flicker, as though being blown by a draught. He had put this down to static electricity formed in his body and being channelled through the pin, like a transmitter. This led to many other experiments later by many other scientists, but none were apparently concerned about the human body's bioenergies; this is a field of endeavours which has been mainly Chinese up to recent times and is another clear aspect of Yin and Yang between East and West.

Faced with the knowledge of the energies, you can challenge people's incredulity, or disbelief if they still do not admit to feeling anything (they must feel something, but might be either in denial or unsure), by asking them if they believe in radio or television. These media factors are nothing but the modulation of electrical energies. Radio waves, for example, are sounds which are picked up by a microphone and then translated into electrical impulses which are processed and then transmitted via an Antenna by: e.g. Frequency Modulation (FM), or Amplitude Modulation (AM). These electrical impulses are channelled down a wire by method of amplification, pushed into an aerial and thereby launched into space to be picked up by a similar antenna and machine at another place. Qi is not really any different, and it can be transmitted from one person to another – as in Qigong Healing. Nowadays many people who suffer from back pain might go out to a Chemist shop and buy a Tens Machine. This small device emits electrical impulses which can work on two basic levels, the releasing of muscle spasms and adjustment of energy channels. Anyone using one of these devices should be a little more likely of accepting Qi as the Tens Machine is just another form of transmitted energy.

Where does Qi come from?
The Universe is full of energies, electrical or otherwise. Not only does energy radiate from the stars (suns), but every planet has its own pulse and there are 'radio' emissions emanating from all directions, some taking billions of years to reach planet Earth. There are invisible forces surrounding planets, suns and other bodies, some more subtle than others. When we are born we are already in possession of our own personal 'frequency' or resonance, and possibly tuned in with that of our mother. Once out of the womb, we are subjected to even more external forces, weiqi as the Chinese call it, Universal Ch'i. Some observers, who became known as Astrologists, noted that humans exhibited traits that could be linked to the movement of the planets within our solar system at the time of their birth. The solar system has cycles, daily, weekly, monthly and yearly. As our solar system spins through these cycles, energy waves are produced and they are almost the same each time – a bit like ripples in a pond, they will be almost identical. Astrologists devised 'birth charts' which

described how the movements and positions, transitions and phases of our solar system may affect a child's personality at the time of birth. Obviously there may be slight variations caused by intermittent factors or odd occurrences. In the West these birth charts are called Horoscopes and Sun Signs.

In the East they have horoscopes too, but these are known as Moon Signs. The Chinese use the theory of Yin and Yang plus the Five Elements or Wuxing, but are best known for their use of animal traits: rat, ox, tiger, dragon, snake, horse, sheep, monkey, rooster, dog and boar; in that order. Being an older culture than ours, they may have learned some lessons from their observations which westerners have not, yet. For example, in Japan a woman would not want to give birth to a child in a Fire Horse year, especially a female child. Such a child would bring great trouble and strife to the family as this sign is not only rebellious but said to be 'out of control', like a crazy wild horse which simply can not be fenced in. From personal experience I would have to say that I have faith in these systems, both in fact. In the field of Sun Signs is a friend of mine called Jane Sunderland. Jane is well known as a strikingly good astrologer. On quite a few occasions I visited her for a tea and a chat. Jane asked how things were and I would describe how my life was going, good, bad or indifferent and when I thought it would change. Jane kept a copy of my birth chart, almost in memory as we are not far apart in birth sign terms. She would then spring to her almanacs and references, saying, "Aha! That's happening because x-planet is here, and such-and-such is in conjunction with...", and I have to say, it was spot on and no other explanation could be found as what I felt happening was accurately described as being "planetary effects" in her voluminous books.

With regard to the Moon Signs, I can only say that I have used one reference book in the main, that of Theodora Lau, the Handbook of Chinese Horoscopes. Another very remarkable woman with great knowledge and highly astute powers of observation. Having had experience with not one but two Fire Horse women (born 1966), I can only say that those two experiences were enough to put me firmly on the defensive and concede to the eastern theories! On other counts, yes,

Theodora Lau's descriptions of basic and complex sign types are uncannily accurate and I have even used these in the past to resolve differences between "warring" personalities in my Club, with great success, I must add.

Remember, we are dealing with energy and its various forms and effects. The Chinese call all energies Qi. However, there is Earth Qi, Sky Qi, Heaven Qi, plant Qi and water Qi, etcetera. Each has a slightly different effect. The point here is that we have these energies going through our body, we may create energies within our body and we also create 'man made' energies that permeate our atmosphere as well – radio, television, magnetic fields, etcetera. When the human (or any other animal) body dies, the energy leaves. Without energy we are dead meat, to put it simply. The finer point being that if we are born in harmony with some energies, contain and create other energies, use these energies to run our personal bio-systems, and can change these energy fields within or around us, then why can we not just accept that we need these energies? Qigong, and indeed acupuncture, yoga, Taijiquan and other Taoist Kung Fu systems, use methods (Fa) to build, balance and harmonise energies. There have been many, many experiments in the far east, it appears, but hardly anything resulting from these has trickled through to the western hemisphere. This could possibly be because westerners are obsessed with the external, machines, gadgets and industry, whereas there is a tradition of Internal Medicine in the eastern hemisphere. Here in the west we need to put more effort into the Art of Life, not the Hi-tech art of Lifestyles.

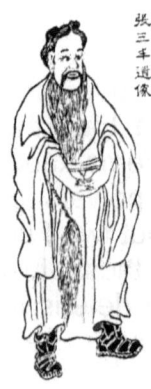

Zhangsanfeng, once a highly sought after government official, gave up his work to travel, learn and study Chinese Arts and became the recognised founder of what we call Taijiquan today; a form of exercise based on strength-building self-defence work which reflects the principles of Taoist philosophy (T'ai = Supreme, Chi = Ultimate and together they refer to the Universe, Ch'uan = Fist/Exercise or Boxing Exercise, together meaning, 'Boxing Exercise in accordance with Tao'). This was an extraordinary accomplishment and one which has positively affected millions of people's lives and is today spreading wider and wider like the ripples on a pond. This is a classical example of Taoist dedication and commitment to one's own beliefs.

It is a common known fact that Earth has a core of iron, a magnetic pole – running from south to north – and many magnetic fields and influences both in and around it, in the earth's atmosphere. It should be no surprise then that humans, like other animals that we share the planet with, use these forces in daily existence.

Personal Enquiry.
Contemplate the above section. Then meditate on how many energy systems you can think of, anything which uses a form of electrical energy, radio waves, pulses, magnetics, household circuits or what ever. You may be overwhelmed by how many there are. What about the Universe, do stars (suns) and planets create or emit energy? Does this create energy fields and are they static or moving? Also ask yourself whether you can accept the theories of Acupuncture, Qi and Qigong which are in themselves based on movements and functions of energy.

How does It work in the body?
Qi is developed in the body as well as being sourced from outside the body. The generalisation of Qi in the body is a bit too technical for me to explain, so I will use analogies. The body generates Qi in much the same way as cars produce motion. We have a fuel tank, the stomach, into which we put food and water. This is processed via our own carburettor, the intestines. The resulting nutrients are then passed through our pipes (the blood vessels) to which ever parts of the body need it most; the body has a wonderful system for healing and building which is governed without our consciousness of it, rather like a self-running computerised control system which neither needs maintenance nor mankind to construct it. Some fuel energy is stored, some is burnt almost immediately, like the process in a car of combustion, burning fuel with oxygen to drive gears, or in our case muscles. We have electrics already, but some is produced by the body (neiqi) whilst we take some from outside (weiqi). Some is used for healing and building, some is used for thinking processes, nervous systems, muscle control and some is used in the general processes of the internal organs and their bio-support – the processes which are 'tuned' in acupuncture.

As in a car, the performance depends upon the quality of the fuel that is put in the tank, plus maintenance. Those people who take their body for granted and neglect the maintenance schedules may find that they start to develop coughs and spluttering, then breakdown unexpectedly. Then they have to call out a mechanic... er, human condition specialist, to fix them and get them back on the road. By eating correctly and understanding what you put into your body (see 'Tai Chi Diet: food for life) you can avoid clogging up the system with trash. By exercising, not drastically, in an enjoyable way like Taijiquan and Qigong, you can keep the system "lubed" and in good working order, including the bio-systems.

Qi in the human or animal body works a little like a complex household energy management system. We have energy for moving and seeing, thinking and acting (lights, tasks and heating), system protection and maintenance (monitoring), power for growing and healing (building and repairs) plus the power to run the power (regeneration) constantly. Humans, being what they are, may tend to overlook the need to be practical and spend all their time doing things which may damage the system, like taking drugs, or sadly in the case of many females of the species, waste what little energy they have on shopping for clothes just to make the outside look good (?) whilst completely neglecting the inside; then wondering why they become ill. Likewise, many males of the human species will eat junk food, excessive meat, smoke or take drugs and again, wonder why they become ill. Strange, but that is life and part of the human weaknesses.

My Oxygen Theory of Qigong.

This is just my theory on the effects of oxygenation in relationship to qigong. Ch'i or Qi works in the body from the inside and its effects spread outwards. Many hundreds of years ago in the Orient, those interested in medical scientific advancements had to do pretty much the same thing as they do today, cut up human cadavers to discover what went on inside. By knowing something of the dead man or woman's lifestyle, work and environment, they could get a good idea of how different tissues should compare; if we think of an obvious example nowadays, such as a cigarette smoker's lungs, then a smoker's lungs would be blackened, clogged up and filled with nicotine tar, etcetera, whilst a non-smoker's lungs would be a healthy purple-pink colour with good porous tissues. One thing that the Old Taoists noticed was not only tissue health but bone health too. They found that the more exercise a person had done the better their bones and 'bone marrow' would be. At the centre of our bones, amongst other repair and maintenance systems, is a function that most people take for granted. This is where the red blood cells or 'red corpuscles' are produced. The red cells are produced using haemoglobin within the main bones and are then fed into the system to replace old, worn, diseased or dead ones. The red corpuscles are responsible for transport in our body, they pick up and deliver oxygen and nutrients to all parts of the body, including the bones. It is, in miniature, like the arterial road services we have in every part of the world; 'red' lorries are built, then sent out to pick up all of our daily requirements and deliver them where needed; at the same time other lorries deliver parts and fuel to the factories where the 'red lorries' are made. Amazing how we copy nature and then credit ourselves!

During the process of Qigong we learn to use the Diaphragm Muscle – just below the Solar Plexus – more effectively. This has the effect of increasing air flow into the lungs. The air, filtered through the nose and warmed on its way to the lungs, travels down the Trachea and then is diverted into the left and right Bronchia which feeds the air into the lungs. However, the lungs are not just empty sacks of skin, inside are three main sections or chambers, the Upper Lobe, Middle Lobe and the Lower Lobe of each lung. The Bronchia (feed tube, in simple terms) then splits off into smaller feeds called Bronchiole, like the branches of a tree. At the ends of these are Alveoli, like small clusters of veins, capillaries and lung tissue (see the illustration below). The oxygen we breathe in passes from the Capillary Network through the walls of each Alveoli and into the

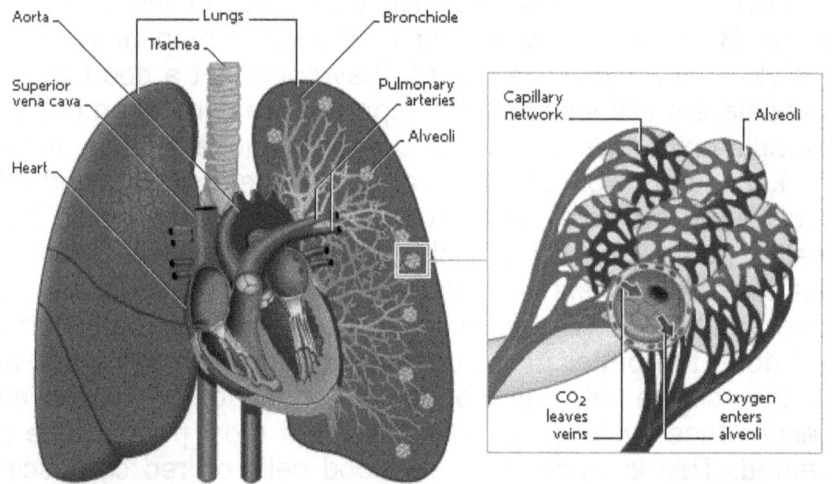

Veins which then pass back out of the lungs and around the body, going through major bones on the way. The oxygen is carried in the red cells to all parts of the body. You can think of it as being a bit like the Underground 'Tube' railway system, the red cells being the carriages and the passengers (oxygen) getting on board at the main station, then getting off again at which ever point they are needed to work at. The oxygen is then used as fuel or in conjunction with other fuels – basic building blocks – for growth, repair and general maintenance of the body.

After just a few weeks of regular practice the Qigong student will begin to notice a few changes to his or her routines. These changes may be subtle, but might include:
- Deeper sleep
- Better energy
- Clearer thinking & improved memory
- Improved libido
- Improved bowel and bladder movements
- Raised appetite.

This is simply because the body, the whole body, has been getting more oxygen and this in turn improves the build quality and therefore performance of every single cell in the body, given time and regular practice: notice that I keep saying regular practice! There are other factors involved in this improvement aspect. One of these is self massage. As the Diaphragm Muscle is used to breathe, deeper breathing means larger movements of this muscle. The Diaphragm is situated just below the heart level, right in the centre of most of the body's major organs. The effect this extra diaphragmatic movement can have by giving a sort of massage to the internal viscera is not only stimulating but health inducing; helping to move fluids, food in the digestive system, bile, blood and much more, so preventing stagnation.

The cyclic effect of regular qigong practice is such that it firstly repairs any weaknesses in the basic system, whilst also developing bioenergies, then it builds up general strength and follows on by making "reserves" stronger and the body more resilient to accident as well as helping improve the quality of the immune system, nervous system and all the tissues that make up our fine and overworked, under appreciated bodies. In other words, the cycle improves and strengthens with practice. In later stages Qigong can awaken and strengthen powers within the body and Mind that most people would probably think impossible in the first place. The reason why so many Taoist Sages live longer than the average person is because they practice daily Qigong, and in fresher air; even those who were told by their doctors when younger that they had some incurable disease and would die by the time they were thirty or forty years old; then by taking up Qigong and perhaps Taijiquan, they lived to seventy, eighty, ninety or even one-hundred.

See under 'Living with Qigong' for some simple Qigong exercises which help sleep, energy, thinking, etcetera.

What about living or working environments, are they comfortable and appeasing? Many Oriental people, as well as Occidental these days, use Feng Shui ("Fung Shoe-ey"), the Art of Divination and Harmonics, to achieve the correct settings. For example, a bedroom which is painted red. This is the colour of fire and is the most stimulating colour in the spectrum. Red encourages activity, but if over used can create anxiety, tension, excitement and headaches or even violence; recall the old saying, 'Like a red rag to a bull!'. Many fast food outlets use a combination of red and orange to promote a feeling of dynamic energy. Violet may be a reasonable colour for a bedroom as it helps create a sleepy feeling, too much though may cause apathy and withdrawal.

The work place is something which most people can not change, whereas the work is. If you are not happy in your job and it makes you depressed, so damaging your health, then 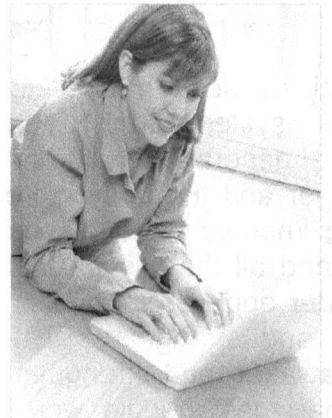 there is an urgent need to change what you do, or where you work. Work should be something that we like doing and not a daily drudge that makes us feel miserable. When helping students with lifestyle issues I have often suggested that they make a list. Divide a sheet of paper into two columns, head the left-hand column 'Likes' and the right-hand column 'Dislikes'; this is so you can carry on overleaf easily, as most people have more dislikes than likes! Over the course of the first day just think about the subject, but list anything which comes to mind – these first thoughts will be the strongest and most important as well as obvious. Then, gradually over the next day or two, add the other likes and dislikes. You will start to build up a picture of your feelings and understand what it is you need to change. You may need to study the list over the course of a few days. Just leave it somewhere safe but noticeable, then pick it up and read what you have written, then let it 'digest'.

Raised appetite is last on the list but not necessarily the last thing you would notice. Food is essential for body growth and repair. Just remember that, as with all exercise regimes, the body needs adequate nightly rest and a wholesome diet, not junk food; what you put in is what you get out.

Many people that I have come across in relation to exercise classes and especially the Chinese Internal Arts tend to fall into one of three main groups:
- Those who do not bother.
- They come, they try, they give up after a short time.
- They come, train, then give up as soon as improvements are noticed.

The remaining few percent are those who make time and realise the importance of regular practice for life, not just after Yuletide! Work, stress, family and studies all play their distracting part, I know, we are all prone to these factors. Often I get students returning to class after a short period of extended work or other problems that "stopped [them] from training" and saying something like, "Oh I felt awful. I had to stop the other day and then I remembered and did my Baduanjin/Taijiquan/Taoist Kung Fu... oh, I felt so much better after that!" The moral of this story being of course, the more often you practice the better you feel.

As humans the hardest task we will ever face in our lives is that of taking control of ourselves. Many people start off with good ideas and good intent but then may fall by the wayside, some sooner than others, some later, some after many years even. However many times you may wander "off the path", know that you can get back on it and reach your goal. Just remember that your goal is long term and there is no hurry, in fact the longer it takes, the better the results will be.

Extending Qi.
After a few years of practice, if you are lucky, your instructor will show you a few Qigong developments, like Qi Sensing or Qi healing. There are many aspects to Qigong that are associated with one of the three main practises, Health Qigong, Medical Qigong or General Fitness Qigong. Then there are speciality fields, like Martial Qigong and Weigong.

Reiki.
Many people in the western hemisphere have heard of Reiki Healing but few have heard of Qigong Healing. Reiki originally came from China, like so many other Japanese practises. Someone in Japan then "formalised" it, formality and ritual being a big thing in Japanese culture but not in Chinese, at least not in the same sense. Nowadays many people earn lots of money from teaching three levels of Reiki, although it seems that the majority of students never go past the first level. Qigong has many facets, amongst these are methods whereby a practitioner can affect the Qi of another person without the use of massage, acupressure or acupuncture, or any other "obvious" act. Perhaps the main reason why the Chinese never formalised any practice like Reiki (Weigong) is that the Chinese people differed in their outlooks on life. In China there was a strong belief that everyone was responsible for their own daily health upkeep, so would practice some form of qigong exercising every day; and when they were lapse, struck by an illness or did not look after their health properly, then they would see a Doctor who would diagnose the problem.

There are many ways of extending or 'growing' your Qigong practice. You can not only learn TCM, healing or therapeutic work, but also take up Taijiquan, for example. There are three types of outcome for those who stay in the Arts, one is healing and the other is teaching, the remainder of people practice only for themselves.

The Meridians and their functions.

The meridians are often called energy channels. Each channel has a specific function or purpose. Qigong and Taijiquan, done regularly, are like battery chargers, they boost the system. The energy channels work separately yet together, if one is damaged it can drain or take power from the other. This is known as 'the destructive cycle'. By regular practice of certain qigong exercises these energy channels can be boosted and "tweaked" for better performance, and with the right combination of foods and exercises the boosting of one can lead to the boosting of the next, and so on. This is known as 'the constructive cycle'.

The Meridians.
01. Governing Vessel (Middle Back)
02. Conception Vessel (Middle Front)
03. Lung (Yin)
04. Large Intestine (Yang)
05. Heart (Yin)
06. Small Intestine (Yang)
07. Pericardium (Yin)
08. Triple Warmer – San Jiao (Yang)
09. Liver (Yin)
10. Gall Bladder (Yang)
11. Kidney (Yin)
12. Bladder (Yang)
13. Spleen (Yin)
14. Stomach (Yang)

Numbers 3 to 14 above are often called 'The Twelve Regular Channels'. The Governing Vessel and Conception Vessel are main functions and can be thought of as master controllers. The San Jiao is not an organ in Western Medicine, but may be likened to functions, rather than tangible flesh. The Lung channel is probably the most hard worked and often imbalanced as this not only relates to the skin (the largest organ of the body) but is affected by emotions and stress as well as outside influences.

The theory behind the formation of the channels stems from the first cell of the body, the fertilized egg cell. When the cell is fertilized it starts to multiply, the first four cells form the upper left, upper right, lower left and lower right parts of the body and like a folded wet painting almost, the meridians are duplicated on each side, one Yin (left) and one Yang (right). The simple diagram below may not be technically accurate, but serves here to demonstrate the effect: The original cell, or egg cell, is number '1'. This then duplicates itself and is labelled '2'. Cells 1 and 2 then multiply again, this time forming '3' and '4'. This illustrates in a very simplistic way, the way in which the human body starts to form. If you look at the 'four cells' diagram, imagine that '1' represents the top left side of the body, '2' the lower left side, '3' and '4' the right side of the body. In Acupuncture the majority of treatments are on the left side of the body. However, the Energy Channels are "reflected" left (Yin side) and right (Yang side): the back of the body is classified as Yin, the front Yang, but this is not a referral of Yin or Yang in the Energy Channels – see below for further detail.

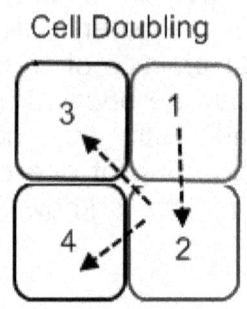

Cell Doubling

The 12 Channels and Flow.
The Qi flows from the upper chest area out along the inside of the arms in the three Yin Channels, Lung, Pericardium and Heart. There they connect with the three arm Yang Channels which flow along the outer aspect, Large Intestine, Triple Warmer and Small Intestine, flowing back up the arms towards the head. At the head these channels connect with the three corresponding Yang (outer aspect) Leg channels, the Stomach, Bladder and Gall Bladder. They flow down the body to the feet. Here they connect with the leg Yin Channels (inside aspect), the Spleen, Liver and Kidney. These flow upwards and to the head and complete one cycle of qi circulation within the twelve main channels.

Each limb has six energy channels, three inside (Tai Yin, Juo Yin and Shao Yin) and three outside (Yang Min, Shao Yang and Tai Yang). By this definition of flow and interaction you can easily understand how the restriction or imbalance of one channel can lead to the weakening of another. On the rough diagram that I have drawn below, the main channels are shown both front and back – bear in mind that these channels are 'reflected' on each side; or in other words, the same each side of the body.

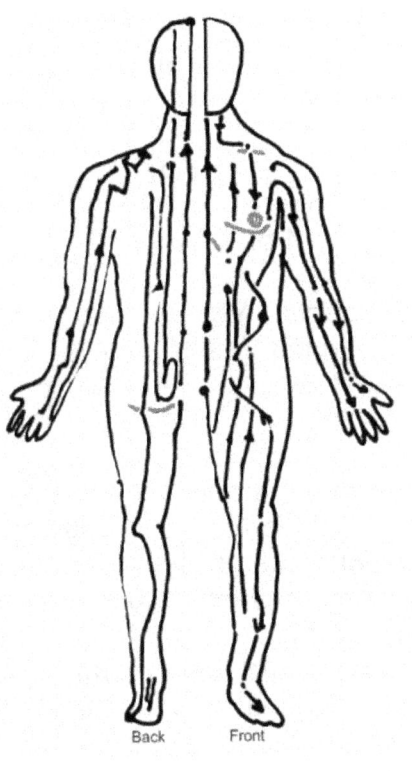

On the right side of the illustration is the Front of the body. The hands and arm are displaying the palm-out position; palm facing you, the reader. On the left side of the illustration you can see the back of the body and outside aspect of the arm. Some arrows have been included to indicate the flow of the channels. On the inside of the leg there are both centrifugal and centripetal (against gravity or outward moving) flows, but on both the Governor and Conception Vessels (central channels front and back) the flow is upwards towards the head in both cases. There are other meridians which have not been included here, such as the Belt Channel, as these are not pertinent to this particular aspect of training at this point.

Bearing in mind what was said earlier about everything having cycles, the meridians or energy channels are no different. The Qi flows constantly through all channels but each may also have a peak time and low time.

Below is a simple chart which describes these peak times and functions. P.E.L. Is used to abbreviate 'Peak Energy Level'.

P.E.L.	STEM	ORGAN/FUNCTION	FLOW
1 - 3 am	Yin	Liver	Centripetal
3 - 5 am	Yin	Lungs	Centrifugal
5 - 7 am	Yang	Lge. Intestine	Centripetal
7 - 9 am	Yang	Stomach	Centrifugal
9 - 11 am	Yin	Spleen/Pancreas	Centripetal
11 am - 1 pm	Yin	Heart	Centrifugal
1 - 3 pm	Yang	Sm. Intestine	Centripetal
3 - 5 pm	Yang	Bladder	Centrifugal
5 - 7 pm	Yin	Kidneys	Centripetal
7 - 9 pm	Yin	Heart Constrictor	Centrifugal
9 - 11 pm	Yang	Triple Heater	Centripetal
11 pm - 1 am	Yang	Gallbladder	Centrifugal

Conception Vessel - Yin - Centripetal
Governing Vessel - Yang - Centripetal
(No Peaks).

When a person becomes ill, there will be imbalances in the flow of bio-energy along one, or more, of the Meridians. At various stages along the lines are points and sometimes the energy may lose momentum and weaken or become 'clogged' by too high a flow. This is when qigong can 'flush' the system and restore the natural flow, if not then a visit to a highly experienced Acupuncturist could be all that is needed to restore the balance. A person who is well studied in the Chinese methods of Diagnostics and Healing will be able to tell, after questioning and examination, what the problem/s may be. Treatment can be had in several ways, acupuncture, Acupressure, herbs, massage, diet, exercise, counselling or some alternative method. There is no "best" cure for any illness or dis-ease, it is purely horses-for-courses.

Modern China is extremely different to the western world when it comes to medicine, although there is sadly a growing dependency on drugs. However, move away from the cities and developed towns and a different story again may emerge. Traditional 'Bare-foot Doctors' still exist in modern China, mainly because the country is so vast, with villages far flung from roads or waterways, that the only way to get there is on foot. The Bare-foot Doctor may use modern drugs, 'sugar pills' or herbs in his treatments, otherwise traditional methods of TCM may be employed. In some villages the traditional herbalist, acupuncturist or other general TCM practitioner can be found. Most Doctors of Chinese Medicine today will use a variety of techniques, including Tui Na massage to treat patients.

In early stages of qigong practice you may not be aware of the flow of Qi, although you may experience strange 'tingling' sensations. It is very unusual for a beginner or novice to be aware of Qi flow in their arms, legs or specific energy channels. In later stages you may feel strong sensations in the hands, especially the palms. Later still you may feel Qi flowing along the arms or the spinal area channels. What ever you do, do not panic or have doubt if you can not feel it at first.

After some years of practice you may be able to not only detect the Qi flowing through the body or limbs but be aware of imbalances too. It is not unusual to find advanced practitioners not only keeping balanced health through regular practice, but diagnosing or detecting early health problems or pathogens and then treating them. Such treatments may include a change of diet or specific food, Qigong exercising or self-massage and acupressure.

Hand Positions in Qigong.
You will see that, for example, in Eight Qi Gathering Breaths, the hands are held 'palms up' as you breathe in and raise them up to head height. This position is used to collect Qi through the hands. As the hands reach head height, they are turned over, or palms facing down. In this position the palms are "guiding" Qi down through the head and body, helping to "wash" the energy channels and increase Qi flow. The hands therefore can both receive Qi and emit Qi. Although this can be done without the hand movements, by using the mind's will to control the Qi, the hand postures are commonly used to both absorb and guide Qi. In healing the hands are used to transmit or express Qi out to a recipient, the "patient" and in China they have actually conducted scientific experiments whereby a

Qigong Master has "anaesthetised" a patient whilst he was operated on. The experiment was very successful and the patient was awake all the time but never felt any pain or discomfort.

Up to here we have learned that external Qi can be gathered through the hands and expressed through the hands. The hand movements work in harmony with the mind to Qi flow in and throughout the body; being distributed via the Meridians.

There is another aspect to what is happening when you use your hands in qigong exercising. You consciously follow the movements of both the hands and the Qi with your mind's eye, therefore you are subconsciously training the Mind to guide the Qi. This practice has an accumulative effect and in time a good practitioner will be able to use the Mind's Will to both gather and express Qi, either inside or outside his/her body. For example, later on in this book you will read about an exercise which gathers and strengthens Qi at the lower Dantian, Expanding the Dantian. This is but one exercise where the hands are not used and the Mind's Will is used to control the energy. There are many other Yin Qigong exercises, some which concentrate on boosting the seven glandular related energy centres, some which boost Qi flow at the main energy channel points or gates. Each has its own purpose.

Qi – Energy.
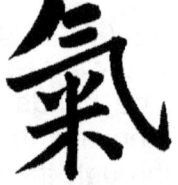
Within the Universe and our perceptible aspects of it here on earth or out in space, as we call it, there are certain forces at work. These forces have both visible and invisible (to the human eye) aspects which manifest in different ways. These forces can sometimes be seen, like the transition from day to night, or from summer to winter. These are obvious. The less obvious forces are often energy sources which may sometimes be felt but not seen. Sometimes we see the end result of one type of energy within our atmosphere build up and release, we call this Lightning. Lightning is one aspect of the Earth's Ch'i (Ki in Japan, Qi or Ch'i in China and Prana in India). Ch'i or Qi is pronounced "Chee", but abruptly, pulling in the Diaphragm as you utter it. For the purposes of this book I use the now

common (but not accurate) modern Pin-yin spelling However you spell it it is still pronounced "Chee". Who has Qi? You have Qi, a Dog has Qi, in fact all living creatures have it, it leaves us when we die. It is part of what westerners call Spirit, but there are many levels to this Spirit of which humans talk, including Mind and Consciousness.

There has been little publicity for Qigong until recent years when Chinese Arts have enjoyed a huge public début, mainly brought about by the US television series of the 1970's starring David Carradine, 'Kung Fu'. This led to many things and many awakenings in the west. Qigong used to be practised by a lucky few, poets, philosophers and lords, but until recent years was not really thought of as public domain material: typical of the Chinese to create something useful and then not make its use widespread – until now.

Since the 1990's there have been so many books written about Qigong that you could easily fill a very long shelf. This has brought with it a deluge of opinion and fact, style and fiction, enlightenment and confusion. Amongst it all are snippets of information, ego polishing, artistic endeavour and many other human factors as well as some very useful information about Qigong. Many books have been written by genuine, experienced and knowledgeable practitioners, some by enthusiastic lay practitioners, dedicated life-long practitioners and developers, others by pseudo 'masters', keen amateurs, etcetera. There are some books written in such a way as to blind the reader with either real or pseudo-scientific terms and illustrations which, quite frankly, can baffle even a long term practitioner of Qigong, let alone a beginner. Let me make one thing clear, or at least attempt to. Qigong is an exercise in which posture, movement, breathing and mental control are combined in certain ways to achieve goals. The 'teacher' need not have a background where a traceable lineage in Chinese Arts is necessary, he or she may have a natural ability which has been honed over the years, they may have a background in Indian, Japanese or even Tibetan studies of a similar nature, or they may have learned from a reputable teacher of Chinese or other nationality. Either way, it is what they know, not who they know, what they can do and teach, not what they can say, the end result being the empowerment of you, which is the most important thing. Following this, my advice is for those who would learn now so that in the future you may help others: study the Art so that you may both feel it and know it personally, do not set yourself up as a teacher – if you are any good at what you do others will call you teacher – nor should you rely upon any claim about your own teacher to prove your worth, just do your best.

Many Ways, One Way.
The development of Qigong, as mentioned above, has been mainly due to Taoist endeavours. Although people who have followed other ways have also developed other similar methods and should not be dismissed. The Taoist methods are in my considered view whole and supreme. How can I justify this bold statement? Simply because the Taoist Arts are whole and complete within themselves, for they range from Qigong through to Taijiquan (T'ai Chi Ch'uan) and many other styles of Chinese Boxing skills (generically Ch'uan-shu, also nowadays Wu-shu), through dietary principles (Ch'ang Ming or Tai Chi Diet) and Taoist Yoga (K'ai Men) right the way across the board to Feng Shui ("Fung Shu-way"), Acupuncture and (TCM) Traditional Chinese Medicine (Trad. Chin. 中医学) and even Chinese Horoscopes. Of course, we must not exclude the philosophy which is the underlying foundation of all these Arts, Tao: the driving power of the Universe and life itself. The philosophy of Tao is a reflection of the governing principles of the Universe and it is these governing principles which have guided the Taoist Sages in their development of Qigong and all the other skills. Of course, sometimes personal influence creeps in, only natural, this is why we get so many variations of one Art. Even in other aspects of Nature we see this; there are more than one species of tree, ape, human, bird, fish or flower. Forget the Henry Ford principle!

The simple truth about Qigong is that there is a "narrower path" of exercise which forms the core of the Arts. Some forms of the Arts can be unnecessarily complicated and references made in scientific terms which may even baffle a well versed Feng Shui Master! Having said that, do not disregard any other form, for once you have learned the basic truths and experienced the power of Qigong for yourself, then you can evaluate other Forms armed with personal knowledge. The methods here are simple enough and if you follow the advice to the letter you should make good progress in your understanding; you need to have the advice and support of a good instructor as s/he alone will know if you are following the exercises correctly. A good instructor of Qigong needs at least ten years experience in study and practice: this is the Chinese 'rule of thumb' for most practises. Understanding of the subject and achievement in it are of prime importance but not in any great depth: e.g. You do not need to understand acupuncture in depth, but a lay knowledge of the meridians and basic functions are helpful. Personally I would recommend that you study this book in conjunction with a well experienced Qigong Master; there are a few about but you may have to travel, the efforts are worth the results. Do not try to learn from a book or even a video with this subject.

Health Warning:
In so-called 'modern' society (although I see nothing different to our society today than what was happening thousands of years ago; Technology is the only thing to have changed.) there is a prolific drug culture. Taking any drugs, be it cannabis or tranquillizers will have a detrimental effect upon your body and its functions. Do not mix drugs and Qigong. Learn to eat and live better before practising Qigong. Change your diet for a healthier one, change your lifestyle for a healthier one generally. Only then will you gain true benefits from the practice of Qigong.

Qigong does have another side, Medical Qigong. At a basic level this can include simple exercises (like Baduanjin) which will increase oxygen circulation, Qi intake and distribution, and also increase blood flow, brain activity, skeletal and muscular strength and flexibility, etcetera. There are also specific exercises for common illnesses or maladies which can be applied by an accomplished medical qigong practitioner.

Anyone with high blood pressure, heart problems, back or knee problems or who is recuperating from a serious illness or women who are pregnant should consult an experienced Qigong or suitable medical health practitioner before attempting any of the exercises discussed herein.

Never practice Qigong when you have a fever or very high temperature!

DO NOT attempt to learn any Form of Qigong without the supervision and guidance of a fully trained competent Qigong Master!

This book is meant to deal with the basic methods for health, simplify and unravel some of the 'mysteries' of Qigong and also provide some insight as to its place in western health and fitness training, sports or other daily activities. This book is a great 'aide de memoir' for those who are studying Qigong or Traditional Chinese Medicine (TCM) and above all it also fills in many gaps left by most training sources as well as dispelling the many myths and avoidance of explanation which can leave one bewildered and confused.

How Should I Go About Learning?

You have bought the book, so you are either an enthusiastic practitioner or a potential beginner. If the latter, follow the advice about seeking a medical health expert's opinion before starting. If you are 100% healthy and are about to begin training, read on.

Most people are unfit, even though they may disagree. The biggest culprit may not be the obvious lack of exercise, but instead may be the wrong diet, unhealthy living or working environments, smoking, drugs (prescribed or not), unhappiness and stress, pollution or many other very common factors of the so-called civilised world. We are not only what we eat but where we live, how we live and what environs we work in. In other words, it is all about "lifestyle". Our lifestyle may need a complete overhaul. Before you go screaming mad wondering about how you start or where you start let me clarify a few invaluable pointers.

Never rush headlong into new ventures. Let the ideas roam around your mind for a while. Weigh up the pros and cons. Do not just throw in your job, unless you have something better to go to; we all need to live and the 'dole' does not allow for that, just a meagre and inadequate sub-existence. An old proverb says, "Every journey begins with just one step". This does not just mean that one step should begin the journey and then you start running. One careful step follows with another careful step, then another, and another, and so on.

The first step however is preparation. Without it you will get nowhere. The first step is the most important. Both physically and psychologically, how we take the first step usually dictates how the rest of the journey will end up, or how long it will last. The better it is planned and the more considered each step is then the better the resulting quality will ensue.

Preparing for Qigong.

Preparing for Qigong is something which you may have already done or there again you may have missed it because you have already started classes and missed proper preparation. Assuming that you have already started let us go through a few essential Way points that need to be ticked off on your journey:

Many people fall by the wayside because they look at the many changes they need to make in their life and feel defeated by the sheer weight of them. Not even the greatest person in the world could change their diet, lifestyle, adopt two or three training sessions a day, adapt their work, clothes and even friends and family life to make way for a sudden change. Each thing has to be worked on and we must take each journey just one step at a time. Remember that well worn saying, "A journey of a thousand miles begins with just one step." Be sensible. Plan. Be positive.

Living With Qigong.

Once you have begun your qigong practice on a regular basis you will notice gradual changes within your self. There may be a few "wobbles" too, like minor acne, sneezes and common ailments, this is just the body getting rid of toxins. This is natural, see the regime through. There is more advice on the subject of practise below, but remember two things that are very important:

- ✗ Never practice anything other than that which you are taught; e.g. not from a book/video and/or without personal instruction. Qigong is something that you can not make up, like a dance routine!

- ✗ Never train with any person who has not enough years experience or who is not a verifiable instructor; e.g. has not trained under an established Qigong Master.

- ✗ If you experience any strange effects or feel ill then consult your Qi-gong Instructor or a Chinese Doctor immediately.

Are You Breathing ?

More to the point, are you breathing as well as you can? Most people are not. Some people tend to breathe from the upper part of the lungs only. In the East they call it "shoulder breathing" as the shoulders rise and fall with each breath. Other ways of part-breathing are "middle breathing", where the shoulders and abdomen are virtually still but short, almost panting type breaths are taken. Overweight people often breathe this way. Then we have "belly breathing" in which the shoulders and chest remain still but the abdomen expands when breathing in and flattens when exhaling. Of all three common breathing methods only the last one comes close to being good for you.

Insufficient oxygenation of the body tissues can have some drastic results. Most of the symptoms would not be noticed at first but would build up over a period of years. Then the problem would manifest after months or even years of almost unnoticeable gathering ill-health. Most people seem to accept illness and shrug it off saying something like, "oh well, it can't be helped I suppose.", or maybe, "we all have to be ill at some time... we can't go on for ever!". This is all negative thinking and there is no purpose served by neglecting your health. Breathing is part of the 'metabolic' system (metabolism: the sum total of chemical changes in living matter; metamorphosis).

The bone-marrow helps create haemoglobin, the red oxygen-carrying pigment in the red blood corpuscles. The corpuscles are pumped around the blood stream by the heart and also carry proteins and nutrients which are processed by the viscera (the internal organs). We only have one heart and it sometimes finds it difficult to pump enough blood to all the far flung corners of the body. The oxygen is transferred to the blood cells as they pass between the walls of the lungs, the oxygen helps to produce better haemoglobin which, in turn produces better red corpuscles capable of carrying more oxygen! If the red corpuscles are inferior and the lungs are not functioning then this all adds to the decay of the system. I mean 'decay' literally as any tissue which is deprived of a supply of essential nutrients decreases in quality and in performance. I strongly believe that 'tissue starvation' is part cause of such terrible diseases such as cancer. Smoking and particularly the inhalation of the "unused" smoke - which is 75-95% of a cigarette and contains over 60 known cancer causing chemicals - is also one of the major causes, plus the biggest drug problem the World has! Smokers are not only killing themselves but hundreds of others. It is mass murder on a huge scale, a holocaust of drug destruction by get-rich tobacco barons!

How Should We Breathe ?
Many years ago the human species generally got more exercise as they had to move camp to where the food was situated, or go out hunting. All labour was manual. This is all exercise to some degree and deeper breathing becomes spontaneous. When you run, cycle or perform exercise sets you automatically breathe more deeply and stimulate the metabolic system. But do not suddenly enter into exercise that you are not used to. As I said earlier, take it slowly, one step at a time so that the body may adapt properly.

On that note it is prudent to tell you that the Forms (Individual Exercise Methods) illustrated within this book are meant to help anyone who has been studying with a qualified teacher. Should you wish to take up proper practice of Baduanjin then I wholeheartedly recommend that you consult our website listing at www.tai-chi-kungfu.com for a U.K. teacher near to you.

Don't cram it!
One of the mistakes that you can make is to force your breathing. You should try to breathe deeply, perhaps more deeply than normal: as you would if you were running or riding a bicycle up hill. Do not try to "cram" your breath in under pressure, or force it, like someone trying to force extra clothes into a case and sit on it. Your lungs are probably not working as hard as they could be, due to being relaxed or lazy in our breathing as well as perhaps not getting as much aerobic exercise as we used to when younger. When beginning Qigong we must learn to use our lungs all over again, but this time "fully".

Always start on the out breath, to clear the lungs so we are not taking in fresh air on top of stale gasses, etcetera. Next, inhale and gently but positively expand the lungs with fresh air and allow the upper part of the chest to expand. Let the middle part of the lungs and rib cage expand (heart and solar plexus level), then finally the stomach and abdomen area as you feel the diaphragm muscle expand downwards.

When you exhale, allow the upper chest to collapse and empty, then the middle area, then the lower area of the stomach and abdomen. Follow through by pulling the diaphragm muscle upwards so that it pushes all the air out of the lungs. Remember, do not FORCE, but do breathe more deeply than normal. If you get at all dizzy, or "oxygen drunk", then relax the breathing until you feel normal again.

**AVOID DUST, FUMES AND
CHEMICAL SPRAYS AT ALL TIMES !**

Try being conscious of your breath while walking, during morning exercise and before going to bed. Use your diaphragm muscle and breathe more deeply, but not strained. Gradually you will feel an improvement and it will become natural to breathe fully. If you study infants or 'toddlers', you will see that they have both good postural and breathing habits. Somehow, sadly most of them will gradually develop bad habits as they get older. Taking in sufficient quantities of oxygen is important in Qigong. Follow the advice on breathing with the instructions for each exercise.

Many westerners make a big mistake. When going on holiday for a week or two they give up practice of their Qigong or other routine, like Taijiquan. Commonly, over eighty percent of these people then feel they have to give up training after their return, because they feel "out of step". This is totally the wrong attitude to have and as foolish as spending money on a new car that will only get used for a few weeks before being left to rot and rust. When you go on holiday, try doing your Qigong before breakfast (after washing, etc.) and you will feel as fresh and as energised as can be. It is really wonderful and can make all the difference to you, even the difference between enjoying your holiday or feeling exhausted from work previous to it. Plus, there is nothing like the experience of doing a beautiful Qigong routine as the sun is setting.

If you experience any strange effects which are not mentioned in this book as 'natural occurrences' then consult your Qigong Instructor immediately.

Preparing for Qigong is something which you may already have done or there again you may have missed it because you have already started classes. Assuming that you have already started let us go through a few way points that need to be ticked-off on your journey:

1. If you have not already done so, change your diet/intake. Eliminate one bad substance from it this week, then aim for another next month and another the month after. This may be chocolate, too much dairy produce, red meats, smoke inhalation or "support" drugs.

2. Look at your environs, at work or at home. What could be done to improve it? Better ventilation, brighter, cleaner, opening spaces, dust filtering, an ioniser (they help most rooms)? Make a plan. If it is at a place of work present it to your boss as a work enhancement plan. Consult with your co-workers too.

3. Be positive; always think of the long term benefits.

There you have three simple things that you can do that will change your life beyond recognition over the course of time.

There is another thing that needs to be done. Research. Reading this book will help. There are many different forms of Qigong, as mentioned elsewhere in this text. If you are in average good health, and wish to maintain or even improve on your health, then practising a Medical Qigong Form will not be the correct course of action, whereas something like Pa T'uan

Chin ("Baduanjin") would be. If you have a Liver problem and have been told you should take up a specialised Qigong exercise to help strengthen your liver, then get expert advice and proper recommendation. Always make sure that what you are undertaking is the correct form of exercise or practice for you and your body.

Finally, but of equal importance, is the need to find a good instructor. Even in China this is not an easy thing to do and just because someone "along the road" holds classes, does not mean that they are the most suitable person to teach you. Traditionally, in many cities in China, people would wander along to a local Park to see the many, many groups of exercise going on there each morning and evening. There will be many Taijiquan Teachers there, plus Qigong and even Chinese Aerobics. There may also be a practitioner of Traditional Chinese Medicine there too, treating people for common ailments. Chinese people are cautious, they may ask for recommendations from students or other practitioners, watch closely and observe, then finally make decisions based on who they thought was a well qualified and respected teacher; Chinese do not take qualification as being a Certificated person who has attended a course, but someone who really knows their stuff! Too often in the West, people pick instructors based on appearance, advertising or even fashion; e.g. just because it is a new group and friends of friends are going to it. If you have to travel, then travel, as finding the right instructor for you is very important and can mean the difference between staying involved or packing up and losing out.

Having done the above you are ready to begin your life-long practice of wonderful Qigong, and reap the many rewards of diligent exercise.

Other Important Factors.
Where you practice is very important, especially at home or work. Follow the basic guidelines below.

- ✓ Home: Make a pleasant and relaxing space. This should be dust and fume free (including chemical air fresheners) with a nearby window which can be opened to let in fresh air. A garden which is not near a main road is also very desirable, especially under a tree or by a moving water feature.

- ✓ Clothes: Wear loose fitting cotton clothing. The cotton soled Chinese shoes (black with white woven soles) are ideal for Qigong, or Taijiquan, as long as you are not on a slippery or highly polished surface. Avoid nylon carpets too.

- ✓ Times: A regular time is best. Early in the morning or during the evening when the air is still and more clean is best. Otherwise, when you can. Make time every day – the results will be well worth putting other things off for.

<u>Simple Exercises.</u>
Do you recall the list of common factors that was mentioned in 'My Simple Theory' Chapter? No? Here is a reminder:
- Deeper sleep
- Better energy
- Clearer thinking & improved memory
- Improved libido
- Improved bowel and bladder movements
- Raised appetite.

The first of the list above, deeper sleep, is achieved quite simply by oxygenating the brain and should be a natural by-product of Qigong practice. Many people do not enjoy a good quality sleep period and feel irritable, tired or lethargic when they get up in the mornings. The body requires between six to eight hours rest each day in order to heal or build; this is why children need lots of sleep to grow properly and usually, or in theory they *should*, sleep between ten to twelve hours each night. Whilst we are asleep there are many, many processes happening within the body, from digestion through distribution, repairing worn or damaged tissues and building new tissues, excesses or waste being taken care of and, if we are lucky, resting.

Sleep quality is improved with oxygenation of the brain and there are Taoist exercises that one can do just before getting into bed that will actually help this process along. Sometimes humans bite off more than they can chew, so to speak, and take on huge amounts of stressful tasks which can cause anxiety, mental hyperactive condition and tension, all contributing to a restless state of mind and making good quality sleep almost impossible. If your sleep is not good then try this simple exercise and affirmation before bedtime each night.

Bed Time Qigong:

1. When ready for bed, sit on the edge of the bed. With your left hand fingers, block your right nasal passage whilst squeezing your arm across your chest – restricting lung capacity. Breathe deeply eight times through the unblocked nasal passage, slowly and deeply.

2. Lower the left hand and arm. Now do the same with the right arm across the chest and the fingers of the right hand blocking the left nasal passage. Eight deep breaths.

3. Repeat steps one and two above.

4. Next cross both arms over your chest so that your hands press on opposite shoulders. Try to squeeze your upper chest area as though restricting the lung's ability to expand the upper rib cage area. Breathe deeply another eight times.

This simple exercise is supposed to gently force air through the lungs because the lungs are restricted in their expansion. Although I doubt that this has been medically tested, it may well have validity, not least of all because you will be taking in more air than usual anyway.

The effects of oxygenation are probably overlooked far too often when it comes to health maintenance and health problems, especially the more serious ones. It would be wonderful if members of the Western medical profession collaborated with members of the Eastern medical profession and Qigong Masters to take the connections many steps further. The future must, and should, lie more in preventive medicine, as it has done for centuries amongst the revered Chinese people.

Bed Time Affirmation.

1. When you have completed your Bed Time Qigong, get into bed and get comfortable; preferably lying on either your back or your side.
2. Know that when you have completed this you will swiftly fall into a deep sleep and awake refreshed the next day.
3. Focus for a moment on comfort. You are snug, warm and relaxed and ready for a good night's sleep.
4. Repeat in your mind, "My body is as strong as a mountain, my thoughts as clear as the mountain stream. While I sleep my body will heal and become stronger." Repeat this at least eight times.

When this simple exercise is finished, in your mind you see yourself as being empty-minded and drifting into a safe, warm and empty black space: this space is created by and controlled by you, so no other effect can enter it, like a protective bubble.

The second effect on the bullet-list above is better energy. This may be something which you are not entirely sure about. The reason for this is that having better energy does not mean that you will be whizzing around like a young child, or that you will be able to stay up and party longer! Having better energy can be subtle. You may notice that you do not feel so sluggish in the mornings, or even in the evenings after a hard day's work. Partially this may be due to being more relaxed too as Qigong has that effect also.

Qigong is a great energy booster and energy leveller, so you may just notice that you seem to generally cope with every day life better after practising regular Qigong. Below is a simple exercise which can boost your energy fairly quickly and help you through those difficult times of the day, or evening, when your energy is flagging.

Energy Boost Qigong.

1. Stand in a quiet, dust and fume free place with clean air.
2. Pull in your lower abdominal wall; hold one hand on the abdomen to assist if necessary.
3. Breath deeply, but not strained, into the upper chest and down to the Middle Dantian (Solar Plexus), so expanding the upper chest but not the abdomen – this is Buddhist Breathing, the opposite to Taoist Breathing.
4. As you exhale, allow the abdomen to relax.
5. Repeat a few times.

Do not use this exercise in lieu of proper rest or refreshment, or good food and good exercise for health. This is only to be used on odd occasions as an energy booster.

Clearer thinking is another effect mentioned in the list above. Because you are oxygenating the brain and generally improving the blood quality and its capabilities, the brain will benefit. Oxygen, as well as rest or meditation, are essential for brain-power. Never take for granted or underestimate the power of breathing correctly, nor the power of rest. All living creatures need rest.

Try one of these simple exercises to improve clarity of thought:

1. Jigsaw puzzles. These can improve your power of thinking and recognition of patterns. Make sure that you are sitting in an upright posture whilst you do the puzzle, so not to cramp the Diaphragm movement. Take deep breaths regularly.
2. Word or Number Puzzles. These can improve brain power and also help in many other aspects of life.
3. Meditations. Taoist Meditations often use Nature as inspiration, like bird song, waterfalls, the rustling of the wind in the trees. You can concentrate on virtually anything. Concentration equates to focus and focus is

an integral part of thought clarity. Sit quietly and concentrate on one sound, then try to hold that sound in your Mind for as long as possible.
4. Reading. Apart from the obvious gathering of knowledge or titillating the imagination, reading improves concentration, logical steps and clarity of thought.
5. Counting. When walking the dog, or taking a brisk stroll between home and the shops, count your footsteps. Buddhist Monks have used this method for centuries to stop their minds from 'wandering' and improve concentration.

a) Counting your breath is a simple Qigong practice. Sit quietly in a dust free area. Exhale. Breathe in to the count of 4. Hold for 1. Exhale to the count of 5. Repeat this without strain for as long as possible; this also has beneficial effects on the overall breathing.

One of the side-effects of practising Qigong, or taking up Taijiquan, etcetera, is that of increased libido. Be wary of this as you can quite easily expend more energy than you create, as well as losing vital stores of proteins and minerals. Taoist Lay Scientists noted over many years and generations, that younger men could discharge their seminal fluid on a fairly regular basis without exhibiting any debilitating symptoms other than the odd bout of tiredness. They also noted that as men got older, if they kept up the same kind of regular ejaculation, they may become more tired or even ill. Hence they eventually arrived at a formula which said that men should lessen their ejaculations as they got older, as well as lessening them in winter months too; the body needs more energy and proteins, etcetera, to get through winters. One of the aspects they did not understand, because of lack of tools to delve further then, was the balance of vitamins, chemicals, proteins and minerals in the diet and within the body as a result. To go into this subject in more depth I refer you to 'Tai Chi Diet: food for life'. Suffice to say here that we now have more knowledge about vitamins, minerals, etcetera, these days and for instance know that Zinc is not found in adequate quantities in most people's diets. This, combined with other minerals, can contribute not only to the production of sperm but also the health of the immune system. Simplistically adding one and one together, it is easy to see that a poor diet could contribute to a lack of ejaculate and poorer health if a man keeps up an active sex life, especially into later years.

Taoist teachings recommend that a beginner in Qigong or Taijiquan, etcetera, becomes celibate for six months to a year. However, if you are married then this may not be practical. In that case take a regular vitamin and mineral supplement which includes Chelated Calcium, Zinc and Magnesium as this will not only help replenish some of the lost substances but also increase the health of the immune system. Selenium is another one, but be very careful not to overdose on this as too much can have a damaging effect. Proteins are essential in the body and you should make sure that you are getting enough in your diet.

After a year or so of Qigong the differences in yourself, or someone else, will be quite clearly noticeable. Added to those bullet-listed points above will be a better complexion (provided the diet is good) and less health problems generally; however, you may notice "wobbles" a bit more as you become in tune with your body. Overall a better lifestyle is achieved.

Improved bowel and bladder movements can be attained by practising the deep diaphragmatic breathing methods. Any movement in exercise will have a strong effect, not only for the bowels and bladder but for all the internal organs and their functions. Qigong, Martial Arts, including Taijiquan, or any movements where you are using the whole body and especially the muscles of the torso, will help improve the movements of the bowels and strengthen the bladder, help the digestive system, improve flow of blood, bile and waste, eliminate pathogens and generally improve the nervous system and other functions.

Appetite is naturally raised by exercise, whether it be by going out for a brisk walk, playing tennis, practising Taijiquan, or what ever. All you need to do is to make sure that:
1. You choose the right kind of exercise.
2. You increase your exercise in regularity and length gradually and under guidance.

3. You eat the right things: expending energy makes the body require nourishing fuel, foods that build, repair and create the right types of energy.

R&R.
Rest and relaxation have already been mentioned enough in the pages above regarding this list of effects. When it comes to rest and relaxation though many people have the wrong ideas, or the wrong settings. Take the subject of beds as a prime example. How many readers will complain that they have a poor night's sleep on a regular basis but then fail to check their mattress, or base, to see if the problem is there? I did this, then went out and bought a 'memory foam' mattress. Problem solved? No. Money wasted! Over the course of the next two years my sleep got worse and worse and I awoke to a worsening back ache too. Eventually, coupled with a very stressful period of family issues, I had to go see a therapist who performed deep tissue massage. She told me that many of her clients who had severe back ache also said that they had memory foam mattresses. This persuaded me to investigate further. The next step was to buy a decent, well known brand of pocket sprung mattress. The difference became apparent within a few weeks.

Pillows need checking too, make sure that yours give you the support that you personally need and that you are not bending your neck whilst asleep; this can contribute to neck ache, shoulder aches and headaches.

Basic Training Methods

Qigong may be done in two ways, standing or sitting still or by moving. In both methods the emphasis is placed on correct breathing formulas and proper mental concentration. In the static form, known as Yin Qigong, one may be lying down, seated on a basic kitchen type chair, seated in a 'meditation posture' or standing still in one of several postures – these are very powerful exercises! In the moving exercises, known as Yang Qigong, the movement is dictated by the need: e.g. Both could be a medical Form or General Health-come-Exercise Form.

"There are no short cuts in Qigong"

Everyone must start with the foundational methods in all skills, here in Qigong it is the correct breathing technique which should be the first step. There are no short cuts in Qigong. There again, the way I teach, Qigong is not that difficult. However, you must allow time for regular daily practice and follow a healthier regime; you can not go out clubbing all night, starve your body of nutrients, eat only sweet or snack foods, inhale or ingest smoke or other toxic drug substances and still expect to gain better health! The human body is a wonderful machine, but it has its limits. You would not treat your car in that way and expect it to last, so you can not expect your body to fare well under such adverse conditions.

Regularity
By allowing yourself adequate rest, eating small but properly balanced meals and using time every morning and evening to practice you can gain fantastic results. Use the time when you would otherwise want to stay in bed that half-hour longer; once you have done your Qigong you should feel like tackling the day head on. Do not collapse in the armchair with negative thoughts every evening, find a nice space, fresh air and do some Qigong, you can find vitality that you never thought

possible. Qigong can change your whole life for the better, your work becomes better, your play becomes brighter and everything else will improve, from your love life to sports.

Almost everyone should realise the importance of regularity. We know that when our daily routines are broken up and made irregular, such as when a baby comes along, we start to feel tired and what we call "run down" - like a clock mainspring or an old battery running out of power. This is also the case when we are confronted with the aftermath of late nights and working days, changes of pace or any other situation in which our body, mind and energies are pushed to extremes. Regularity is the key to good health and success. Looking at life from a Taoist perspective, regularity is a part of Nature. We have days, nights, seasons and cycles everywhere. The whole Universe is going through cycles. On a more personal level, our heart has regular beats, our bioenergy goes through cycles and women of course are all too familiar with the monthly menstruation cycle. Therefore, having learned a lesson from Nature, we can be healthier and happier if we have a regular pattern of rest, fuel intake, work and study, plus our maintenance schedules, like qigong or meditation, of course.

Overall Qigong is a simple yet wonderfully effective method of gaining a better energy with stronger healing powers. It has often been incorporated into other Arts and given odd or gimmicky names, but there is only one Qigong, Chinese in origin but of use for anyone, anywhere in the Universe. There are of course different schools of thought relating to Qigong methods and practises. I was reminded all too sharply of this when watching a popular TV show where a presenter was looking at different Martial Arts around the world. An ill-informed commentator spoke of a Japanese Karate practitioner who could paralyse someone by using a Ki-ai/Qi-hai ("Chee-aiy") or Spirit Shout. He said that there was no relationship between this and Qi, and that the Chinese were in "disarray" regarding Qi. This is not only inaccurate but an ignorant statement, it was way off the mark. The Chinese were the first to recognise Qi and it was they - more specifically Dr. Hua, To – who discovered and developed Acupuncture and other aspects of Qi and Qigong which are recognised world-wide today. If my memory serves me well, it was Donald F Draeger, a man who studied many Martial arts systems in the orient including China and Japan, and he commented something to the effect, "The only things that the Japanese have invented for themselves are inter planting rice with barley and a storm lid on a lantern. The rest they have borrowed, mostly from China. They are like the magpies of the Orient." In fact, Karate itself derives from Chinese Crane Style Kung-fu, via Fukien Province to Taiwan, then Okinawa before Japan where the partially learned system was relabelled as Kara-Te.

The Chinese have some very well developed systems of Qigong and it is the more highly developed and popular exercises that I concentrate on. From these have sprung a selection which are compatible[2] and can be used, as needed, in daily life without too much concern.

Many people in the West are unsure of what Qigong is or whether they themselves should try it. To give perspective and place to it below you will find a brief comparison of popular sports and exercises with their good and bad points highlighted to the best of my ability and experience. Experts in each endeavour will of course be able to tell you more.

---

[2]Compatible exercises are important. Each method can set up its own pattern of energy, like magnetic fields, vibrations, impulses, etcetera. Most Qigong exercises for daily health practices are amplifiers and levellers of energy within the bio-system, therefore reasonably safe. Some exercises can focus or drive Qi to specific areas or create fields of energy which may imbalance an otherwise fairly well balanced person, thus causing ill health. Thus in T'ien Ti Tao P'ai only compatible health exercises are taught generally with specific Qigong only being given to those who need it at the time and self experimentation is discouraged.

How Does Qigong Compare with Keep Fit, etc.?

There is a common misconception, centred in the western hemisphere, that fitness is something to do with muscle tone, stamina and being thin. This is not fitness, this is simply the result of someone who burns off more calorific content than they intake, at the same time as working the body hard, and often to extremes. The Chinese – who have studied exercise for almost five-thousand years – call this Wei Kung, or 'External Training' and someone who builds muscle is likened to an Ox. Western fitness studies and techniques are in their infancy. Would anyone in China pay a Personal Trainer to go jogging, cycling or 'do weights' with. Not likely. Why? Because the Chinese culture has studied many aspects of health and fitness training for hundreds and hundreds of years and they would look at this practice with amusement and bewilderment. The Chinese methods of health and fitness are far longer developed and far surpass anything in the West.

Around one in one thousand Personal Trainers can sustain their exercise routines after the age of forty-five, one in two-thousand after fifty years. People in their sixties and seventies can take up or continue their Chinese health practises and enjoy the benefits way into later life. This knowledge is widely available in China – and is now becoming more widely available in the western hemisphere, but awaiting western awareness and acceptance to catch up. Obviously there are some differences and those have to be catered for. For example, in China most people realise that they are responsible for their own health. If they do not know how to gain good health or maintain it, then they will go to a suitable person to learn from. In the West most people are still in the habit of relying on other people to maintain their health, whilst they might continue in negative lifestyles, depleting their health again. Personal Trainers and Coaches may be necessary, but these should be suitably trained people who do not concentrate just on external appearance and calories, but on educating trainees how to eat, exercise correctly and even breathe correctly, as well as maintain health for the long term. This is where Qigong comes into a world of its own.

If you were unwell or unfit in China it is most likely that your Doctor would spot the area of health and fitness lacking, then recommend you to go to the best teaching source in your area. This might be specific, like Taijiquan, or Qigong, or it might be a trip to a Healer. Either way, Personal Trainers do not exist in Traditional Chinese Culture because Chinese people prefer to get the knowledge from a good instructor in a public class and then make time for their own home study and practice. Having a Personal Trainer in Chinese culture means that you are blindly following someone whom you do not really know, have no idea whether they really are qualified and if they are doing the right things for you personally, whereas in a public class one can see other people who are training with the teacher, ask them questions and see the results for themselves: in the west, weight loss seems to be the prime goal of training for many, not complete health, so training may be imbalanced and dangerous in the long term; western fitness training can have a 'boomerang' effect, for once someone becomes tired of training or can not afford Personal Trainer or Health Club fees, they lessen or stop training and their weight suddenly piles back on; this effect is caused by the 'burning calories mania', if the person focussed on correcting their diet, then taking up regular exercise classes 'Chinese style' and also practice at home (goal setting), the results would be deeper reaching and longer lasting. Another ill-effect of sudden physical training can be the strain placed on joints, like hips and backs, which can become manifest as arthritic and rheumatic disease after long periods of jogging or other physical training. Most western exercise coaches seem to be prefixed on the outer body, whereas most eastern gurus start on the inside of the body, then work outwards.

Overweight People & Underweight People.
There are two main categories of people who are able to participate in Qigong Therapy, 1: Fit, 2: Unfit. The fit person may be free from Cancer, Heart troubles and is not Obese: in obesity there may be restricted blood vessels, weakened heart

or other serious internal organ problems which need to be looked at more closely. Dietary changes are a must to get an obese person back to a stronger state of health. Those who are not obese or suffering from serious illness can take up some form of qigong but should consult a Chinese Physician before doing so: by 'Chinese Physician' it is meant in the sense of TCM, a traditional practitioner who understands these matters. Obesity is sometimes caused by glandular problems, but more often than not just eating too much of certain foods, quite often at the wrong times, and not getting enough exercise to burn off the excess. This needs to be addressed before taking up Qigong otherwise you may not get the desired results.

Underweight People.
Being underweight is also a problem, especially if it is deemed to be anorexia – self-starvation, regurgitation of food, or smoking to suppress appetite and skipping meals. Do not be afraid of food or putting on a few pounds/kilos. Body weight does naturally fluctuate from month to month, so don't panic. What you need to be concerned about is being underweight. Again a visit to a competent physician should put you in the picture. You need to know what your 'ideal weight' should be and then have a look at your diet to see how you can achieve this. Women in particular should not focus on dress size and set goals accordingly, generally speaking anywhere between size 10 and 16 is "normal", so concentrate on healthy diet, lifestyle and balance.

In any case, if the above problem/s concern you then counselling may be a good idea. Anyone with weight problems may have some issues on their mind which need to be talked through with a neutral third party. Sometimes, just by talking about a subject, the person being counselled will find answers to their own questions or problems.

Inside Out.
Western exercise, as said above, concentrates on burning energy to 'tone' muscles – muscles do work more and become

'toned' but become more visible due to loss of fat under the skin. This affects the outside of the body visibly making the person look leaner and more athletic. Invisibly it affects the heart and lungs, the cardio-vascular system. It makes the participant feel better and 'more alive' mentally because of the boost of oxygen to the body and brain. This is good. However, there are and can be many negative side-effects[3]. One of these is joint wear and joint or spine 'compression'. When someone runs there is impact, this happens from the feet, through the ankles, knees, hips, spine and even head. The better quality the shoes the less the effect may be felt, but it still happens. In the long term this can lead to all sorts of debilitating problems, from painful foot conditions (I can vouch for that!) to arthritis of the hips, knees or spine. On a positive note, scientists have found that ".... long-term mild regular jogging, which did not influence either body mass index or maximal O2 uptake, appears to improve insulin action in both carbohydrate and lipid metabolism and to increase the metabolic clearance rate of insulin. " (Researchers: Oshida Y, Yamanouchi K, Hayamizu S, Sato Y.) which could be good news for Diabetics or Hypoglycaemia sufferers, but this is not yet fully proven and one would need to consult medical experts before commencing any form of physical exertion! Note the researchers' use of the word 'mild' in reference to jogging.

Hooked!
One of the factors often overlooked when dealing with exercise and its effects on the human system is 'addiction'. Running, cycling and other aerobic type exercises will burn fat if done for long enough, will increase stamina and will leave the doer with a feeling of well being, of sorts, but these forms of exercise can also be addictive. Many people nowadays have heard the expression, 'Adrenaline Junky', but there is more to it than getting hooked on an Adrenalin high every day. The human

---

[3] A report by Prof. Elizabeth Gould (Harvard University) suggests that jogging could be bad for your health, especially if you do it alone. A team of researchers said that going for a run on your own is not as healthy as people believe. Their research showed that jogging as part of a group is healthier. The experiments they did on rats showed that running alone raises stress levels and slows down brain cell growth.

body produces many different hormones and chemicals to get us through every day life. Some of these are short-lived, some build up in the body and others can have addictive side effects. Another problem is the mind. Often a state which is induced physically can have a mentally shifting state. In other words a person can actually get hooked on extreme exercise, or any activity which further induces the well-being feelings, etcetera. This is the point where exercise takes a swing from being 'normal' to 'abnormal'.

In the UK there are hundreds of Fitness Trainers and Personal Trainers, a percentage of these fall into the 'normal' training category (they train regularly to maintain health but do not over train). A more worrying percentage seem to train far too often, their training becoming their life and taking over from normal issues to the point of becoming an Obsessive Addict. This can be described as a mental health condition known as Obsessive Compulsive Disorder: The diagnosis of OCD is valid only if an obsession and/or compulsion causes marked distress, is overly time-consuming (More than 1 hr./day/session up to 2 sessions, say morning and evening), or if it significantly interferes with normal routine, work, family or personal relationships. In the case of someone who takes aerobics classes every day, does other exercises too, runs for an hour or more each day and appears to be overly concerned about their health and weight (especially when they are of slight build), might indicate serious mental health problems which are being 'buried' under the excessive (OCD) training programme. There are even some who may start to believe that they are Superman, or Superwoman, and feel that they are superior to other mere mortals. A drug is a drug is a drug is a drug. Anything which is addictive is not healthy. If the effects of this are transferred to family, especially children, then a chain reaction of physical and mental health problems takes place.

Below, in the brief comparison, you may note that many western external fitness methods drain the internal resources. In Traditional Chinese Medicine terms, this can have a life shortening effect - as opposed to life lengthening, like Qigong. Many people start out in western fitness looking healthier and slimmer, but soon start to look prematurely aged. Why? Could it be as the Chinese doctors have been saying for centuries, that training externally neglects and drains the internal? Exercising should be balanced, like all things in life. Yin and Yang.

Kids and Exercise.
Children should not be made to exercise excessively, especially any exercise which may 'impact' the joints or force them the wrong way. They should not "do weights", as this will not strengthen them but will have an adverse effect on their bones and joints. Children definitely should not be put on any ultra-low-fat diet. Their bodies can process and burn fat very quickly (up to 30% in daily diet – see book, 'Tai Chi Diet: food for life') if they are normally active children. If they are inactive, then walking, climbing and general play should be encouraged as this will burn off any excess naturally. They should not be put through army style disciplines or adult routines.

Generally children are active. If they are not, and are overweight or inactive, then their diet and lifestyle should be seriously looked at along with the rest of the family's attitude towards food, exercise and lifestyle.

Over Exercising.
Question: "What about Chinese who practice Ta Lu or Martial Arts' Forms for hours on end each day?"
Answer: "This is not obsessive, but necessary. Training always starts with smaller sessions and the practitioner is built-up, slowly. Chinese Wushu Kung Fu or Quanshu ("Chew-aan-shu") Forms are very long and complex. It can take as long as six months or one year to learn a 40 Step Form, then it will still need lots of 'polishing' to get it right. There are foot positions to consider, knee positions, body angle, elbows, shoulders, hips, waist, head, fists, etcetera, plus a host of other elements to do with tension or relaxation, the mind, areas of focus, etcetera. During this process the learning of long sets has a strong and beneficial calming and organising effect upon the brain. A dedicated practitioner will develop higher consciousness, as well as being super-fit and healthy. Much of the learning

process can be less demanding physically and more demanding mentally. Therefore this practice is far removed from the almost mindless practises of jogging or weight training and uses the whole body, unlike running, etcetera. Excessive 'aerobic' exercise can lead to Kidney and Spleen Qi deficiency and illness."

This may pose the question, "What is healthy and where does addiction begin?" Healthy is jogging (or brisk walking mixed with other types of varied exercise) for up to one hour per day, two hours maximum if more complex: i.e. Includes a specialised routine for specific training. If a person is training for a special task or job (e.g. Commandos) then that training may be extended: but not necessarily remain 'healthy' – even tough Commandos suffer from many injuries, after all, they are "expendable personnel" in the end.

Normal exercise is and should be a preventative, reducing risk of pathogens and increasing body functionality, flexibility, etcetera. Healthy exercise does not have to be aerobic or excess calorie burning. In other words, what ever you do or do not do, you eat what you need and no more; humans are like other animals, opportunistic hunters, if there is food there then the psychological need for survival switches in and whatever there is will be consumed, in case there is a shortage tomorrow; in modern societies there is no shortage tomorrow and this overconsumption leads to obesity and other health problems.

Unhealthy is where the activity (usually focussed on one main activity) takes over from normal life and the addict becomes obsessively focussed on it. The 'addict' may then reach his or her physical limits and start finding the need for boosters, like so-called 'energy drinks' with high amounts of caffeine or glucose in them or other Adrenaline highs. Lack of the chosen exercise can lead to depression, or feeling unsettled if not participating in his or her activity. There are large and largely unexplored minefields of mental and physiological as well as physical aspects which, as yet, have not been looked at in enough depth.

Pregnancy.

Most of the Qigong in this book is quite suitable for women under normal circumstances. During pregnancy changes occur and there must be precautions so as not to separate the developing baby from the womb prematurely, therefore many stretches and vigorous movements must be excluded.

Exercises which may be done include:
- Zhanzhuang – Post Holding (up to 20 minutes).
- Eight Qi Gathering Breaths (8 Breaths, any time of day)
- Baduanjin Form 1 'Two Hands Push the Sky'
- Baduanjin Form 2 'Separate Heaven & Earth'
- Baduanjin Form 4 'Horseback Archer'.

NOTE: the Baduanjin exercises must be done gently and the pregnant woman must not over-stretch! Repeating each exercise 8 times is sufficient, but this can be done morning, noon and night or before bed.

The exercises will help the breathing whilst in labour, which is no longer taught by Midwives in the UK, for some strange reason. The qi benefits both mother and baby.

After childbirth the mother needs to regain her energy and rebalance her body. This should begin with at least two days rest while she also comforts and feeds the baby who is also in need of adjustment to the bright new world! The Zhanzhuang or Post Holding exercise can be done lying down after the first day or two of rest. Later on, abdominal breathing can be added to rebuild the strength of the abdominal wall muscles, pelvic floor muscles and other core muscles.

Be Whole.

The Chinese approach exercise (generally speaking) in a manner which is different. The objective is 'balance'. A holistic approach which encourages the individuals to discover more about themselves and their lifestyle. The individual approach ranges from wanting to be a healthy person, to wanting to be a very healthy person. A person wanting to be healthy should look at their diet first. Then their lifestyle: do they exercise, if not take up some form/s; if they do, is their exercise the right form?

Overweight people would obviously benefit from the correct diet (fat limiting) and exercise (depending on heart conditions, etcetera.) to suit their goals.

Underweight people might also want to consider their diet (body building foods) but also those types of exercise which increase body size or bulk: not restricted to weight training by any means; weight training can be detrimental to young people and some others.

The Chinese have known for centuries that the regular practice of Taijiquan can either ward off or reduce the effects of age, arthritis, diabetes and many other common illnesses born of imbalance. Qigong can also have similar effects, but based upon the theories and practices of acupuncture meridians and energy flow, Qigong exercises can also be used in a medical context: this also means that one should be careful about mixing different types of Qigong exercise without qualified (by that I mean highly trained and knowledgeable) instruction and supervision. Generally speaking, it takes a year to learn a set of Qigong exercises, like Baduanjin, fully, then a further year or two to polish up and get familiar with the extended versions. It can take between six months and a year for the Qi to change and develop in the body to a settled state. Learning to become a competent teacher is a matter of practice, firstly alongside an experienced teacher. Becoming an experienced practitioner who can recognise symptoms and recommend particular exercises is another matter, this could take between ten to twenty years; depending on frequency of practice and experience.

Knowledge.
Any activity starts by looking at the subject. Before any action of a physical nature is taken one needs to take a mental approach by understanding what the programme is that you are about to embark upon. Know the basics, understand the approach and the correct method for preparation.

- Study the chosen activity. Try to get different views.
- Understand the correct entry procedure, warm-ups, etc.
- Take it one step at a time and you will make better progress later on – conversely, rush headlong into it and you will fail.
- Monitor each level and your progress.
- Try to understand any errors and why they happened.
- Make notes, keep a Training Diary – what you did, when, how long for, how you felt then and the next day, diet, etc.

The fourth item, monitoring your level, is not essential but is quite useful, especially for those who want to teach later. Being able to see, feel and understand what changes have been made in your body, mind and activities is quite enlightening and empowering.

Understanding errors is essential. We all learn from mistakes. The most common mistakes made in qigong are rushing, not practising frequently enough and doing exercises wrongly. Only with the latter can it be detrimental to your health, and this again emphasises the need for a good instructor.

BASIC EXERCISE COMPARISONS

Aerobics.
This usually conjures up images of girls in an assortment of impractical 'fashion' garments thinly disguised as work-out clothes, with red faces and sweating profusely whilst they jump on and off plastic steps or dance with weights in their hands, etcetera. In fact, aerobics is any activity which makes your heart pump harder and therefore increases lung activity too – cardio-respiratory exercise. Included activities are (what I call) 'pump-and-jump' aerobic type classes, cycling, running or jogging, swimming (fast), brisk walking and martial arts-based exercise, like Kick-box (non-contact).

Good points:
Aerobic exercise can strengthen the cardio-respiratory system, burn off excessive fat and/or unused calories, add tone or strength and stamina to the muscle groups used (mainly lower body in most activities, except swimming and kick-box, or aerobics with weights). A session of forty minutes[4] (intermediate) to one hour (advanced), three to four times per week can leave a healthy person feeling very positive.

Bad points:
Aerobic exercises in a class-based environment can have detrimental effects to the ankles, knees, hips and spine – possibly neck as well. If the venue is air-conditioned, then dust may be an issue with the lungs. There may be problems with Obsessive Compulsive Disorder sufferers, or those with poor diets and anorexic problems. Beginners may be forced to keep up with the more experienced. Many a modern Club Fitness Trainer only trains for around six weeks before being let loose on the public, so therefore have limited knowledge and virtually no experience; if they work in a health club or gym, they may

---

[4]beginners should be firstly trained in diet, then induced slowly with stretches, gentle warm-ups and slowly increased aerobic exercises from periods of five minutes and increasing, depending on health condition to start with.

also pick up habits from colleagues. Others may train weekends at home or at a YMCA to do a short course.

Tip: if you see a Fitness Trainer who drinks caffeine or 'energy' drinks and lives on 'pump action' adrenalin, 'fast food' and tuna sandwiches, then forget it, go elsewhere!

In Cycling of course we would think that nothing much could go wrong, apart from crashing into a large vehicle. One of the more popular health club activities in the 2000's is called 'Spin'. In this a number of people gather on fixed exercise bikes and are led through a fast paced routine by an eager instructor. The bad points to watch out for here are: equipment not adjusted to personal height or pedal reach – knees must never be straightened as you reach full downward stroke (bursitis potential) and the seat to handlebar positions should be adjusted to avoid neck or back strain and of course heart attack.

An instructor in a club or class environment who is taking a "push" based (aerobics) class may not be able to see what is happening to each individual, nor help individuals. Therefore classes can be dangerous.

Body Building & Weights.
Body Building is a bit of a two-sided coin. On the face of it you have those who believe that large muscles and an oversize physique are attractive, and the flip side is for those who consider themselves too skinny and just need to bulk up to a more reasonable level. The latter is understandable, but the former I find bewildering, unattractive and abnormal as there is absolutely no need for it.

Weights are a different thing if used wisely. The most common use of weights in the world is within a purpose built Gymnasium or sports facility. Usually the person follows a set routine, one which has not changed much for many years. The purpose most people apply to weights is what generally is called 'toning the muscles'. There are other more specialized uses, the most obvious being in physiotherapy to rebuild muscles that have lost size and strength due to illness, etcetera. In China, for hundreds of years, people have used weights on a more practical level, to build muscle strength for specific tasks, such as physical labour or Wushu. The kind of weights used differ in this instance as they will use rocks, concrete blocks or large metal implements or heavy metal weapons.

Good points:
Weight training can be very beneficial if done correctly with supervision from an expert; by 'expert' I do not necessarily mean someone trained by a weight lifting organisation, as I have seen such people doing exercises which can be dangerous for the spine (e.g. A concave spine whilst doing high lifting), I consider an expert to be a person with practical knowledge and awareness of anatomical health and is more concerned about health than how great a weight can be lifted. Combining weights with exercise, such as Wushu Kung Fu can have very beneficial results if done correctly; for health, fitness and musculature, not just looks.

Bad points:
There are too many specifics to enter into here. The main points to be wary of are that weight training done incorrectly can put a strain on the spine (vertebra and inter vertebral disk) causing possible leaks or ruptures later on. A less common concept I have observed is that most trainers do not consider the wider picture. When you use weights you put tension in the muscles, causing them to become shorter, tighter and bulkier. The picture above shows one of the many ways *not* to lift weights if you wish to avoid injuries. Without proper care poor practice can have a detrimental effect on the connecting tissues, the ligaments and fascia tissue which 'take the strain'. Weight training, in any form, must be done in conjunction with stretches – warm-ups

and warm-downs – for the affected areas. Children especially should not be encouraged to use weights without the previous point in mind. Children are growing, therefore any tension placed upon the muscles and ligaments can have a detrimental effect on their growth, as it can cause deformation of bones and joints.

Core Conditioning.
This term is used to indicate any form of exercise which publicises itself as strengthening or developing the 'core musculature' of the skeletal system or its stability: this includes the pelvic floor muscles and all those around the lower back and stomach areas which actually hold in the internal organs (the 'corset muscles', as I call them) as well as helping spinal strength. Core exercises have become a bit of a 'hip word' in recent years (AD 2000 <) with many 'wannabe' trendsetters jumping on the proverbial band wagon and developing new routines with large financial gains at stake: the USA, UK and Europe have seen a large increase in the numbers of people, skilled, semi-skilled or virtually unskilled, setting up exercise routines for profit – selling to large fitness clubs or organisations.

Good points:
Exercising the core support muscles is, or should be, an essential part of any exercise routine. Women who have been through pregnancy will know of the effects when their core muscles get stretched and elongated. It can be quite difficult to get these muscles back into shape, especially for women over twenty-five and those who are not fit or inclined to exercise on a regular basis. Most of the core exercise routines I have seen and spoken to trainers about seem to be taken from established exercise systems, such as Taijiquan (Tai Chi, as most uninformed people call it) and Yoga or even Qigong. This poses the question, "Why bother with new Core systems when you already have proven established ones?" Most forms of yoga are excellent for core strength. One Qigong exercise which many try to emulate and often get wrong is 'silk reeling', a basic exercise of Taijiquan. In Qigong there are many exercises which affect these muscles and improve their

strength or efficiency, and even in Wushu Kung Fu, with many more beneficial effects added. So why bother with just a fractional exercise? Maybe the answer lies within the useless human trait of following fashions and trendiness.

Bad points:
Partially covered above. If an exercise is developed by someone who is not fully trained or cognisant of potential injuries, then there are clear dangers. Something I became aware of and was alarmed by was the fact that in health clubs they send one, rarely two people off on a one or two day workshop to learn these new routines. The workshops may hold up to sixty or more people (impossible to check all at all times for correct procedure or safety) and are usually fast paced. The attendee is then awarded a 'pass' qualification (I have never heard of someone being failed) and released to teach the said new form straight away. Often the person or persons who attended, then teach junior staff the new form, warts and all. During this process many of the exercises, postures and methods will get changed along the way: this is inevitable and I can vouch for every other Martial Arts and Fitness Instructor that I know of in saying that we spend most of our time correcting mistakes which have crept into student's Form due to personal interpretation, lack of awareness or just plain forgetting or missing the point. Be warned, be wary.

All Instructors should demonstrate at least three times, get the class to follow, then at some point walk between group's members and correct mistakes. Health Cubs are guilty of the worst offences and should have beginners classes where all beginners are taught new exercises safely and gradually before being allowed to progress to a more energetic or faster paced level.

Dance related.
Dance or dance related exercise is a great way to improve your circulation, stamina and overall ability. It is also a great social pastime and can relieve stress, be fun to do and fairly cheap to participate in. It is not a method of fitness training unless it is mixed with properly thought out and planned

exercise to improve flexibility and muscle tone, etcetera. Of course, some dance styles already contain high levels of fitness training incidentally, like Latin and Modern, but only a fool would jump straight in with poor fitness levels, bad joints and weak muscles!

Good points:
Dancing can be gentle and relaxing or hot and steaming with lots of sweat and body flexing, lifting and fast paced movements. Choose a milder pace to begin with, then look for what you like and what suits your body and health: e.g. If you have a heart condition it would be unwise to go from unfit to Latin, without at least consulting a good physician! Dance can be fun and it is one of the few activities you can share that enjoyment with because of having a partner. Rhythm is good too, you can choose your pace (anything from Waltz to Rock) and stick to it. One of the best things about dancing is the social factor, you get time to meet and talk to new people and enjoy exercising even more that way.

Bad points:
Unless one is unfortunate enough to get a dance teacher who tells you to do something really stupid (e.g. Do something to put your back out), then I really can not think of anything. Flamenco concerns me somewhat, as the heels are continuously stamped on the floor – with or without matting – and this could lead to heel, knee, hip or even back problems later. Another thing to be careful about is bending one's spine over backwards, especially when done suddenly or one is unfit.

Kick/Box exercise.
This regime is usually based upon a mixture of Martial Arts training techniques, Western Boxing and general routines for cardio-vascular fitness. The classes vary greatly in content and quality depending on the instructor's background and studies. Being involved at National Level in the Martial Arts world allows me to have seen everyone from the unqualified, to the low level 'one grade wonder' or the 'Studio Queen' who has never done any in-depth Martial Arts training, or much else, and right up to high standard Martial Arts or Kick-boxing

(fighting variety) levels taking up these kind of classes for the public consumption.

Good points:
Generally speaking this can be a great way of getting fit, loosing weight, gaining strength, focus, awareness and stamina, etcetera, but it all depends upon the instructor and his or her background. Classes can contain a mixture of stretching, general cardio-vascular exercise and coordination work, like using focus mitts or other unfixed equipment.

Bad points:
Torn muscles or ligaments, back injuries, dehydration problems and poor techniques are all unfortunately common problems. These problems come from instructors who either have no proper training or have some training but lack knowledge of how to avoid these issues. As with any exercise class, you are best advised to seek a trusted professional opinion about suitability, and at the moment that is not commonly available, so proceed with caution and common sense. The best way to avoid injury is to understand which exercises or techniques are responsible for causing damage and which are not.

Jogging & Walking.
Walking is natural, it is what humans are [almost] designed for. However, there are more factors involved than just using your feet. Walking is a low impact aerobic exercise and is beneficial to most people who are lucky enough to be able to walk. There are variants, like walking uphill or walking downhill, smooth ground, rough ground and even soft sand. All of these can have different effects, both positive and negative, on the human body.

Jogging is a form of lower speed running which is supposed to be kept at a manageable pace and prolonged for up to forty minutes or more to be beneficial in burning off excess fat or unused calories as well as toning the legs, thighs and buttocks. There are specific techniques to Jogging which should minimize risk of foot, ankle, knee, hip and spine impact and problems later in life. Both joggers and runners may also experience some side-effects of the stomach and lower intestines, they may get more frequent urges to excrete and the stools may not be 'normal' but loose instead. There may also be other digestive disorders, sickness, etcetera. Do not take drugs for these symptoms, change exercise routines instead, or at the very least add qigong to strengthen the internal organs!

Running is more of a specialized sport and the two basic types are track and field, these may include hurdling in the former and hill climbs, or obstacles in the latter. Not only expert advice is required for these but appropriate and correct footwear (specifically for you and your foot shape or foot problems – see 'Bad Points'), advised by a specialist.

Good points:
Jogging can burn off excess pounds/kilograms of fat which is the result of overconsumption of foods (not just fatty foods); the body converts unused calories (food energy measure) into fat and stores it, usually around the waist and hip area. If the metabolic rate is low, this remains unused – the human digestive system is a little like the Camel's hump, which stores water for later use, if we do not use all our food then some is stored as fat – eating lots when food was plentiful, at harvest time, is a natural animal trend and is designed to put on some fat to protect against the winter). Benefits are only noticed when a level of thirty minutes raised and sustained heart rate is achieved, then excesses of fat or calories will start to be reduced; time needed, between forty minutes and one hour for best results – with full warm-ups and warm-downs needing extra time.

Bad points:
Wearing appropriate shoes is essential – especially if you have low or flat arches, over-pronation, etcetera. Likewise for jogging or running. Seek foot care specialist advice. Wrong techniques or unsuitable shoes can lead to joint problems in later life such as arthritis. My biggest concern would be the pressure and shock placed on the legs, hips and spine through short-stepping or jogging movements, which is where the

routine gets its name from as one "jogs" up and down. The heart is our most essential organ. Look after it, improve its strength but do not overwork it. Many people have suffered heart attacks whilst running, and especially Marathon Running, even those who apparently thought that their heart was healthy before taking up the sport.

Many people take up jogging or running with little knowledge or without a medical examination. Advice is simple here, get a full medical examination and expert heart test, expert advice and seek out the proper footwear (suitable for your feet and posture) and always start gently and in the correct manner (walk, jog, walk, jog, walk, stretch out at the end). Personal Trainers and Gym Trainers should be wary and enforce the above rules and make certain that their clients get full testing and purchase the correct shoes. Personally, I would prefer Power Walking to Jogging, but have also learned the hard way that in this activity the "digging in" or high pressure planting of the heels on the pavements can lead to a painful condition known as Plantarfasciitis.

Yoga & Stretch.
Yoga is a terrific form of exercise. There are however several mainstream forms of yoga to choose from. If you are starting out, then start at the bottom (Hatha) and work your way up. Traditionally, Indian Yoga is taught in levels, with Hatha Yoga being the basic level (relating to Earth), then rising up through the levels of Water, Fire and Air to Spirit. There are many schools and each varies slightly, some are combined, so this description remains brief and generalised. There are also many a 'self-taught' yogi out there who in the main teach a hotchpotch of exercise, not all yogic. If you wish to study and practice yoga properly then find a properly trained instructor.

At its most basic level (Hatha) yoga works on the muscles and skeletal system. As one progresses (Pranayama, Rajah, etc.) it involves breathing and consciousness. Meditation aspects are a bonus at all levels and the calming effect on the mind is desired by many in today's stress ridden society; hence yoga's world-wide popularity, especially in stress-ridden western cities.

Good points:
Yoga tones muscles and makes them and ligaments stronger, more elasticated, joints more flexible, aids circulation, improves core strength, mental calmness and regulates breathing in higher levels. Regular sessions of two to six a week are most beneficial.

Bad points:
There are a number of unqualified teachers who may mix-and-match various levels of yoga with Taijiquan, Qigong and even general keep fit exercises. Whilst this mix-and-match is not generally of major concern wrongly practised postures and techniques is and can cause injury (muscle strain, ligament strain) and other health problems. Qualifications are not always standard and not widely used. Some qualifications may be lacking in modern health and safety awareness and not taking into account such matters as back problems, dangers of holding breath and joint forcing. Be aware, ask questions and do not ever 'jump in the deep end', always seek a carefully led beginner's group by someone who explains each yoga exercise and walks around to check individuals as she or he teaches.

Qigong.
There are many forms of Qigong, as you will discover partially from reading this book. Each individual exercise, or Form, was developed for a specific need or reason. Some methods were taken from work or trade skills as it was noticed that these movements had beneficial health effects on the practitioners. Exercises such as Silk Reeling, which came from that work skill, is one. Chinese Punt Rowing is another. Many others have been developed by Taoists who have dedicated their lives to the practice and study of such Health Arts, others still by Martial Artists who have noticed the beneficial health effects of certain movements or postures.

There is no doubt in my mind that qigong can have beneficial effects for absolutely everyone. In its various guises it develops the natural bioenergies and Universal energies that we use in daily life. Those people who are healthy and fit (note that I put health before fitness) may take up any form of qigong exercise which is designed to maintain and regulate the system. Those who need a more specific form, due to illness or imbalances, may require one of the other methods. From time to time we all get a health wobble, a pathogen, which left untreated may cause more serious problems. It is then we need to consult a more experienced practitioner who would be able to recommend the correct course of action – this may be dietary, exercise, environment or medicinal, as well as qigong, and if he or she was unable to administer that correct treatment would know of someone who could.

Having studied qigong methods alongside other forms of exercise and fitness, my personal Qigong favourite has become the New Standardised (& Safer) Eight Strands of Silk Brocade, or Baduanjin. This is an excellent set of exercises which offers a seated version for the lesser able, a standing version for the stronger, and a more advanced version which can add extra benefits for practitioners after a year or so of regular practice. On top of this, the exercises can be used in a more external or physical sense as a pretty good warm-up routine. The health benefits are astonishing and practitioners all swear by it as a regular daily exercise.

Good points:
Qigong can correct imbalances and eliminate pathogens. It can help arthritis, stress, high blood pressure or many other common ailments. The standing postures are beyond the belief of the unenlightened as they develop huge amounts of internal power or bioenergy, fitness and strength. The skeletal frame and the muscles are all beneficiaries, and even the skin (the largest organ of the body) will show signs of improvement too – hence the old saying that Nei-gong or 'Internal Training' reduces ageing effect.

The moving exercises can channel the Qi through specific meridians (energy channels) and can have a pronounced enhancement upon the practitioner's overall health. There are also benefits for the mind and spirit. Many of my students have heard me say that the beneficial side-effects of Taijiquan and Qigong could fill a book by themselves!

Bad points:
Westerners have to accept what millions of Chinese have known for years. There are the good, the bad and the indifferent, even in China. Some methods may have been created in a hit or miss fashion, others by years of medical study, more still through qigong study and re-design. Qigong can and should be a "horses for courses" practice and advice really should be sought. If taught incorrectly, it can lead to imbalances as it may adversely affect the rhythms or cycles of the body's bioenergies or lead to pathogens. Be wary, always seek an instructor who has trained under the direct supervision of an experienced instructor or who is acclaimed by students and those he or she has helped. This type of skill, like many, can not be picked up from books or videos. Personally I know of an untrained couple who used to run public classes and many of their students became ill. One time they dropped in to one of my Baduanjin groups, asking me if it was all right to have a go (Quote) "...as we have been trying to learn it from a book, but was not really sure how the moves go?" They had already begun teaching it to unsuspecting members of the public before they came along to my class – I gave them warnings about safety and health practices and the need to learn properly, under supervision, and just hoped that they would go away and reconsider what they were doing; better to advise people like this rather than reject.

N.B. Martial Arts.
Advice and information found in all the above sections covers most of Martial Arts classes too. There are many styles, some more external, others more internal.

Avoiding injury is paramount, so avoid excessive contact, forced stretches, joint forcing or elbow and knee locking-out. These are just some of the problems to be avoided – especially for children. Full Contact blows or defensive Blocks may cause blood clotting, so if anyone has potential problems in this area they should not take up contact sports.

Beware of any class which has many injured students. Always seek a well qualified instructor and make sure that they are insured and nationally recognised.

Internal Vs. External Exercises.
What the Chinese call Internal Exercise is the exact opposite of External Exercise. Internal exercise involves a formula of integrated breathing, posture and mental awareness or control. External exercise may seem to have the same qualities, but it differs. Internal exercising is practised for health reasons whilst external exercises are often practised for appearances.

Regimes such as weight-lifting, running, Hatha Yoga, External Martial Arts (Hard Style), Aerobics and Dance-based exercises may produce an attractive looking body, at least from the outside. This achievement is often at the cost of the internal aspects, like depletion of the organs and vital substances. This can cause premature ageing, illness and internal weaknesses. The internal organs or 'viscera' are responsible for all daily health, repair and upkeep tasks. The strains placed on them by participating in regular external exercise can deplete them drastically thus negatively affecting the body's ability to regenerate, fight off diseases and strengthen necessary biological functions. Think about a simple analogy, work, rest and play. If you do too much work, or work and play, you know that you will become ill. Rest is important, why? Rest enables the vital organs to use the vital substances for building, repair and maintenance, as well as keeping the immune system and other functions operative. If the vital substances are depleted then no amount of rest will help. Balance is required between internal and external exercising.

Dr. Stephen Chang says, "The internal organs do what thick muscles can not do: protect the body against age and disease. The Internal exercises, in turn, protect, heal and energise the internal organs". I say, "What is inside comes outside". The Yellow Emperor called qigong 'Yang Sheng Shu' – Tao of Revitalisation. These methods date back over thousands of years. Ask yourself sincerely why this is so, why qigong should flourish this long, and take your time thinking about it too;

never form opinions on a one-sided view, so why not try some qigong for yourself for a few months before forming any opinion based on external training?

Summary
The internal organs actually make the rest of the body. If you neglect the care and maintenance of these for the external muscle appearance then do not be surprised that your health will suffer, you may age prematurely and also deplete essential energies and nutrients required for major organ functions!

Personal Trainers, Football Coaches, Athletics Coaches, Weight Trainers and especially School Physical Exercise Instructors need to wake up to the dangers of physical training without internal protection and strengthening exercises – Qigong. The history is there, the proof is "in the pudding", as we say in the West, and there are many hundreds if not thousands of people who can not continue external training into later life; or who have sustained irreversible and debilitating health effects from what the Chinese call 'External Training'.

On the reverse side take a look at the thousands of Asians and Caucasians who practice Qigong Therapy into later life, look younger, stay healthier and stronger.

The obvious aim of this book is to provide some practical information regarding Qigong and its factual structure. One of the other aims of this book is to try and provide impartial advice regarding training, from a pragmatic viewpoint; I hope this works! When it comes to taking up training then this is a two-sided affair where the student seeks instructions and the instructor advises and looks after the student. Below are some factors to consider for both students and instructors. There may be other things that you can think of, questions which could be asked, but for now this comprises a reasonable starting point.

General Advice for potential students of all disciplines is to check out the class instructor of Yoga, Aerobics, Kick-Box or any other, before starting. Every instructor should carry and be able to produce Professional Liability Insurance (a certificate which names an insurance company and policy with a policy number) that shows the expiry date. Many 'Fitness' policies carry Public Liability for students of the named instructor, but in Martial Arts students need to be insured separately as named individuals. It is important that you do both check insurance and make sure that you are personally covered; just think of how expensive health care is now and imagine how you would cope if you had an accident which left you unable to work or pay the bills, how would you cope? Insurance is there to protect the public (you) as well as protect the instructors, as they too could lose their livelihood, house, savings and more, if they were not insured but found liable in a claim or action against themselves.

Most instructors carry a leaflet which explains the history and background, disciplines studied and/or achievements, but nowadays this sort of information is more often than not contained on a Website. Websites are a very useful source of information, and of course, you can do lots of research on the Internet about any subject, sport or discipline you fancy; but do not expect every scrap of information to be one-hundred percent accurate or unbiased!

Qualifications vary greatly, from the traditionally trained long term apprentice who has been made-up to Instructor by his or her Master's approval, to the formalised course with a certificate at the end. Good judgement is needed here as well as perhaps some background knowledge about the pursuit you are interested in as well as any traditional or national training or governing bodies. Overall though the best qualifications any instructor can have after this is the positive feedback from his or her students; if they are progressing, happy and training injury free, then there is every chance that you may be happy too.

Instructor's Advice.

Novice Instructors may not have spent adequate time learning about preparing class routines or training schedules. Therefore I have decided to cover the basics here, both as a guide for the newer teacher and a guide for the public too.

Preparation & Procedure:
- PREPARE room for SAFETY and COMFORT.
- ASK if anyone has INJURIES or PROBLEMS.
- WARN all about over-exertion or STRAIN.
- ADVISE beginners to do less than the experienced members.
- START with stretches for muscles and ligaments.
- WALK slowly around the class to check for bad spine posture, etc.
- BUILD UP slowly and SPEED UP gradually.
- ALLOW rest or SLOW DOWNS between stamina exercises.
- DO NOT let people gulp cold water when thirsty – SIP!
- EXPLAIN what exercises are, how they are done and safety.
- MONITOR individuals who appear to be struggling[5].
- AVOID any exercise which puts strain on the spine or joints, forcing them the wrong way – especially young people.
- ALWAYS warm down with more gentle exercises and appropriate stretches to relax the body.

These are only the basics which need to be remembered for all types of exercise classes or instruction. Programmes generally vary from system to system, level to level. Instructors should be able to design a individual programme suitable for all levels and ideally have separate beginner's classes or induction courses if possible. A Qigong class may attract a wide range of people from the healthy to the unwell, a questionnaire should be filled in before they join and the Instructor/s should know about any problems and understand personal needs.

---

[5]Do not be afraid to ask someone who is struggling, or who looks like they might have a heart attack, to slow down or even sit out if necessary. This is professionalism and client care as it should be.

Avoiding Injury – Important Advice.

The very first stage in avoiding injury is to realise how fit or unfit you really are. It is not possible here to give precise examples for everyone, so here is a generalisation or two. If you have not been exercising, performing a physically challenging job (e.g. Building work, box shifting and stacking, delivery work, etc.) and have put on weight then there are some basic clues there already. Can you touch your toes? No, then your muscles may have 'shrunk' and you are not so supple any more. Can you climb 21 stairs quickly without getting breathless? No? Then you have lost much of your aerobic capacity. Do you spend most of your day seated or hardly moving? Yes? It is obvious that someone meeting this description needs more exercise, but how should they begin?

Self-knowledge is the first step, as outlined above. Know what you can and can not do. As we say when taking exercise classes, 'Know your limitations!' As I write this, being in front of the computer for around forty minutes, I feel the need to walk around, maybe go outside and stretch, or even do some Qigong.

Having taken 'Tai Chi for Health' classes at a Health Club for a few years, I have witnessed many people who are very obviously overweight, and others who's unfitness and ill health were not so apparent, joining up for fitness facilities. New members to the club underwent a 'fitness test' and had their blood pressure taken, along with other basic checks, like weight, heart rate, etcetera. However, they were then given, what I would describe in my opinion, as a 'whistle stop' tour of the gyms and equipment, the guide pointing out small plaques on the sides of fixed weight equipment saying to them, "this gives you instructions if you need help". They were then virtually left to their own devices. Many a member expressed their anxieties to me about being left alone, some were quite scared, but being a 'freelance instructor' it was not something I could or should (for legal reasons!) do anything about. On a couple of occasions I left my group with one of my trainee instructors while I went to find a member of staff for something, only to find one girl on reception and others having a break or nowhere in the building to be seen on either floor or in any of the public places. I know of two men who died of heart attacks in the same 'health club', one swimming and the other doing a 'spin' (cycle) class. On another occasion a freelance Personal Trainer told me that he had to clear the training floor areas when a fire alarm went off, because he could not find any staff available or a Duty Manager! Many of the staff were very young and trained up over a period of just six weeks or so before being let loose on the public. To my mind, the implications of starting training in this way are horrific. These tales alone scare me, especially as training in the Chinese Health and Fitness Arts takes a bare minimum of five years to get to instructor level, and then the trainee is still under supervision.

The only way to approach training is the safe way. Follow these simple guidelines if you suspect that you are overweight and unfit and want to take up some form of training:

- Get an appointment with your Doctor, get weighed, have your blood pressure taken and get an overall assessment of your fitness levels, joint and ligament flexibility and ability to take up your chosen fitness activity.

- Do some research. Find out what kind of exercise you need first; e.g. Stretch, weight loss, stamina, or a combination. Consider walking instead of driving, taking the stairs instead of the lift, and of course, eating a healthier diet.

- Next you need to find a suitable local instructor. Looking in the phone book, library ICON database, posters in clubs and halls or schools will bring up a whole range of activities. Look for experience, qualifications and insurance.

- Asking is the next step. Ask if you can watch. If the answer is 'no' then go elsewhere. Politely ask the instructor about his or her experience and where they trained, how long for, how many years experience, whether they are insured for Professional Liability and

Public Liability, if you can see their certificates or any written history. Also talk to a mixed range of students and ask them about what they do, like or dislike, if possible.

- An instructor could offer you a free sampler session (if a group activity) to see whether you like the activities or not. During this, your first session, warm-ups should be explained or you should be watched and guided on posture and performance: e.g. Tuck your pelvis in, keep your spine straight, do not overdo it at first, etcetera.

- Beginner's classes or exercise sessions should concentrate on quality, not quantity. In other words, you are not going for gold, or for 'the burn' - a sign of very bad practice! Coming out of a beginner's class with a red face, breathless and feeling exhausted are not good signs. All beginners should be induced slowly and carefully, building up pace as they get more fitness and stamina.

- Progress is another key factor. Exercise levels may start off gently but as you progress you can feel 'stagnant', so a change is needed. This should be in the form of exercises or techniques which 'advance' in a natural way, hence taking you from level one to level two and so on. Be careful not to go too far or too fast, or get into the 'adrenalin junkie' trap!

- Nutrition is another important factor. You need to understand your diet and what food does for or to you (see author's book: 'Tai Chi Diet: food for life'). Making sure that you have both energy and body building foods is important. Two hours should be allowed for digestion before training, more is preferable for larger meals.

- Rest is another factor. After exercise rest is needed for the body to be able to 'repair'. Repair includes building, or rebuilding. After exercising muscles and joints, the body sends messages to the brain which then assigns various body functions to build and repair the muscles, ligaments, bones, etcetera, with the elements gained from your dietary intake.

As a generalisation, food, drink, exercise and rest should be balanced to the degree that you neither feel too tired nor have excess energy (hyperactive). If you are flagging and feel in need of 'energy drinks' or boosters, like caffeine, then you have a problem, simply put, you are overdoing it. Eat properly, rest properly and exercise in accordance with your ability and spare time. Similarly, if you are eating too much, resting too much and feeling like the proverbial 'couch potato', then get your days organised better to increase exercise and achieve a better balance. There is no excuse for imbalance or bad health. It happens, but we all have a responsibility to ourselves to look after our health. Work is the biggest excuse for running ourselves into the ground. The work will still be there tomorrow, and the next day, and the day after that. Take a break, do some exercise.

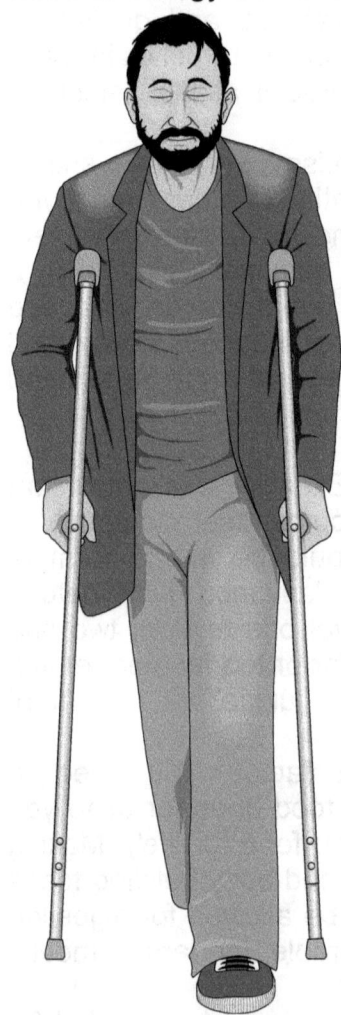

Be Aware.
Some exercises can place tremendous strain on the body and cause 'wear and tear', as the common expression goes. This in turn can lead to debilitating joint problems, arthritis and worse. Problems like these do not appear overnight, they appear in later life – as many hundreds of thousands of 'middle aged' or older people can attest to every year – and more increasingly, younger people too. Ankle, knee, hip and lower back problems are much more rife than you may think, and many of these can

be associated with poorly led exercise classes, too much running or jogging, or other exercises which put terrible strains on the joints or back. One of the most common scenarios that I have come across is that which can be labelled, "The Arrogance of Youth"! You can tell someone who is young until you are quite worn out, about the dangers of certain exercises, but most will still go ahead anyway. Why? Because they can. Because they can not feel it right now. Because most young people are oblivious to the fact that they are getting older and that their "super fit" and capable body will wear out faster if abused!

Thankfully, there are not as many things to worry about in Qigong practice as there are in jogging, football and other exercises or sports renowned for injuries. Qigong practitioners just need to be aware of forcing the spine the wrong way, ridding tension and following the correct advice regarding practises. This may explain why Qigong is so very popular with the Chinese, wherever they may be. It is not my intention to scare the reader away from any exercise which is less than gentle. My intention is to illuminate the many potential dangers which lurk in the field of exercises that are unchecked, badly taught or taken on by well-meaning amateurs who do not know the correct facts and methods of avoidance. For now I will rest my red flag waving arm before it gets too tiring! Think SAFE.

The Basics of Qigong.

There are three basic postures involved in learning Qigong. Each of these may be used according to needs: note the word 'needs', not preferences, for preferences make humans tend to veer toward lazy.

POSTURE 1 – Lying Down:
The practitioner may be weak, ill or infirm and having to spend much time in bed. This posture eases the strain on the whole body and thus allows concentration.

Use a thick rug, foam mat or cushions upon the floor. Lie on one side and bend the knees for stability. Rest the top arm along the side of the body with the hand resting upon the hip area. The lower arm should be bent with the hand, palm upwards and open, in front of the face. Relax and be comfortable.

It is also possible to use the normal lying posture, flat on your back, hands by sides and also palm-up, one pillow to support neck. The problem is that this position can make it too easy for the practising person to fall asleep, so the above posture is preferred marginally.

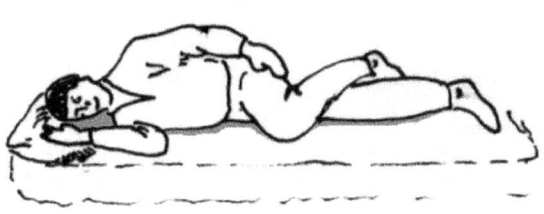

POSTURE 2 – Sitting:
This posture is ideal for anyone who has problems standing for any length of time. It also encourages good posture when seated. Use a normal dining chair, one that allows the body and thighs to be at a ninety degree right angle to each other.

Sit in the chair but do not rest the spine on the back of the chair. The feet should be a natural distance apart and flat on the floor. The torso, thighs and lower legs should be at ninety-degree right angles to each other. The hands rest upon the thighs, just above the knees. Keep the head suspended, as though held up by an invisible string, but without tension in the neck or shoulders. The eyes gaze at the horizon.

POSTURE 3 – Standing:
In the standing posture maximum effect is achieved by adding cardiovascular effort (e.g. the heart is pumping against gravity, but without other physical strain) and the legs and back are strengthened at the same time.

Basic Standing Posture. Stand with the feet shoulder's width apart. The head is held upright, as though supported by a piece of invisible string – Tip: imagine that your frame is like one of those medical skeletons, supported from the middle top of the skull (upward arrow in diagram indicates this upright "pull"). The knees are very slightly bent and the pelvis is tucked in, that is to say, tilted forwards very slightly. This has the effect of straightening the spine. The shoulders are relaxed and hands allowed to hang effortlessly by the sides, although not touching. The eyes gaze at the horizon; as indicated in this illustration by the arrow pointing straight ahead.

These are the three basic postures of Qigong practice. The Standing Posture should be used by all who are reasonably fit and without arthritic leg conditions, sore feet or other debilitating conditions. Even those who are fit and able to stand may find that standing is quite tiring at first, especially when standing still. Never try difficult postures until you can manage the basic postures with ease. Practice will improve this, both in terms of physical ability and concentrating.

Comfortable Clothing.
All cotton clothing is ideal, such as a cotton Tee-shirt and cotton or cotton-based trousers. Avoid Nylon and other man-

made fabrics which can disrupt your Qi flow and cause some strong "static" effects. If you wear loose fitting clothing you will feel and be more able to sit comfortably and without restriction of movement, blood or Qi. Obviously it should go without saying that the general atmosphere should be comfortable too, not too warm, not cold or draughty, neither too bright nor too dim, just 'pleasant'.

Basic Breathing Techniques.
There are two categories of breathing when naming a person's breathing method, shallow or deep. Deep breathing is quite rare, unless exercising vigorously, even then the breathing may not be complete.

Shallow breathing may be split into sub-categories:
- Upper Chest
- Lower Chest/Abdomen
- Middle Chest

In Upper chest breathing the person's shoulders may rise, the upper chest or rib cage may rise slightly, but the middle area and lower chest and abdominal area remains almost motionless. Many hyperactive people breathe like this.

In Lower Chest/Abdomen breathing the 'belly' area will be seen to rise and fall whilst the upper chest area remains almost still. Many overweight people breathe like this.

In Middle breathing, the central area of the chest may be seen to expand, but there is little movement from the upper and lower areas mentioned above. This is often associated with short and slow 'panting' breath, commonly seen in heavy smokers and people with serious lung problems. All three ways are bad for the body, including brain activity, as insufficient oxygen will be taken into the system.
In Buddhist activities they normally teach Upper Breathing, to increase energy quickly and oxygenate the brain for clearer thinking. In Taoism we practice Full Breathing, this uses all three sections of the lungs and chest, including the abdomen.

More on this below. This method too increases mental clarity, but also improves overall health, especially long term.

Insufficient oxygenation of the body tissues can have some drastic results. Most of the symptoms would not be noticed at first but would build up over a period of years. Then the problem would manifest after months or even years of almost unnoticeable gathering ill-health. Most people seem to accept illnesses and shrug it off saying something like, "oh well, it can't be helped I suppose.", or maybe, "we all have to be ill at some time... we can't go on for ever!". This is all negative thinking and there is no purpose served by neglecting your health. Breathing is the most important part of the 'metabolic' system, the heart working with it to distribute the oxygen around the body to where it is needed. As said earlier in this book, the blood does not only circulate the oxygen but all the nutrients too. Hence you can see the close dependency between lungs, blood, heart and digestive system.

Don't cram it!
One of the most common mistakes that you could make is to force your breathing, or strain. General advice is quite simple, you just need to read this and be clear about what it means. You should try to breathe deeply, perhaps more deeply than normal: but not laboured, as you would if you were running or riding a bicycle up hill. Do not try to "cram" your breath in under pressure, or force it, like someone trying to force extra clothes into a case and sit on it. Your lungs are probably not working as hard as they could be, due to being relaxed or even lazy in our breathing as well as perhaps not getting as much aerobic exercise as we used to when younger. When beginning Qigong we must learn to use our lungs all over again, but this time more fully so that we can improve our overall health.

<u>Beginning.</u>
To begin with, use one of the above postures. Get comfortable with the posture. Make sure that you will not be disturbed, switch off mobile phones and house telephone, if possible,

otherwise stick a thick cushion over it and let the Answer-machine take any messages!

At first, be aware of your breathing, 'listen' to it, feel it, know how you breathe normally. Now is the time to make any adjustments to your posture, if not upright, or surroundings if they are distracting or dusty. You must be content with your place of practice and time – this is your special time.

The Full Breath.
Always start on the out breath, to clear the lungs so we are not taking in fresh air on top of stale gasses, etcetera. Next, inhale and gently but positively expand the lungs with fresh air and allow the upper part of the chest to expand. Let the middle part of the lungs and rib cage expand (heart and solar plexus level), then finally the stomach and abdomen area as you feel the diaphragm muscle expand downwards (dotted grey line in diagram). If it helps you can place one hand on the lower chest at heart level and the other on the abdomen allowing you to feel the expansion and contraction of the rib cage and diaphragm muscle.

When you exhale, allow the upper chest to collapse and empty, then the middle area, then the lower area of the stomach and abdomen (solid black line). Follow through by pulling the diaphragm muscle upwards so that it pushes all the air out of the lungs. This whole technique is like a wave effect. Remember, do not FORCE, but do breathe more deeply than normal. If you get at all dizzy, or "oxygen drunk", then relax the breathing until you feel normal again.

Women and Abdominal Breathing.
Many women find that attempting abdominal breathing is quite difficult. This might be for different reasons. One of these may be psychological, as women are generally slaves to fashion and trends, they may be made to feel insecure about their figures by skinny fashion models, advertisements for lingerie or body products and even music idols and film stars. The idea of having to inflate the abdomen, even if temporary, can give some women too much emotional trauma. Obviously this is something which should not occur, but it does. The only way around this is for the woman with these psychological problems to either try self-help or professional help to overcome any fears or preconceived ideas. Abdominal breathing is quite natural. Women with babies should look at their baby and see just how natural it is, female babies breathe this way, it is *natural*.

Another reason might be tight clothing, especially around the waist area. If a woman is not adverse to abdominal breathing, but finds her clothing uncomfortable and restricting, then the simple answer is to replace that clothing with garments that are (a) loose fitting, and (b) made of cotton. Think about traditional clothing in places like China, then you will see the sense in it.

Exercise and diet might be a third reason. Many women these days eat no breakfast, then only have yoghurt and fruit for lunch, and maybe a small meal later on. This is madness and very unhealthy, but can also cause abdominal tightening, irritable bowels and stomach cramps, amongst other symptoms. On top of this, exercises like Sit-ups, will tighten the abdominal muscles. Combinations like this can cause discomfort or even pain if trying to extend the diaphragmatic muscle downwards and expand the abdomen. In cases like this, good health through correct full breathing is going to be much harder to achieve. The first goal is to correct the diet, one step at a time, eating a full breakfast, energy lunch and smaller dinner; or alternatively, full breakfast and then 'snack' all day. This needs to be backed up with a more holistic exercise regime and re-education regarding the female image; women are not fashion icons, not all women are skinny and being skinny is not an element of attractiveness – unless you are very shallow of course!

This may sound harsh and even critical, but it is factual. Fashion and trends, starvation and physical self-abuse have never created a person who is admired by millions! Traditional Chinese Qigong, like many other of her traditional Arts, has deep roots in culture. Chinese culture is threaded with many strands of Confucianism and in this philosophy 'society' came first, so one would strive to make one's self a useful person, a truthful and respectful person, and respecting yourself is part of that. The threads of Taoism are also prevalent, this aims for being natural, not a slave to fashion or minor trends. Taoism also strives for higher levels of health and fitness through naturalness. In Buddhism too there is no place for falsehoods, fashions and self-deception; e.g. thinking that by starving yourself you will become more attractive, or by following fashions and clothing trends. There is an old saying that the poison of Yin is more powerful than Yang's medicine. To a degree this is true, as every day, all around us we can see useless fashions and trends not only ruin the West, but now catching on in the East and ruining some fine old cultures; extremism is not desired either, as it is an imbalance, a balanced person in modern society tries to become more natural whilst using those tools that are available.

Myth: Abdominal breathing makes you look fat! Nonsense indeed. Abdominal breathing, using the Diaphragm fully, not only enhances the overall health of the system and body, it strengthens the abdominal muscles, the pelvic floor and all the essential support muscles (core muscles, to quote a trendy phrase!). Abdominal breathing is great for the female figure as well as health.

Consciousness.
Try to be conscious of your breath while walking, during morning exercise and even before going to bed. Use your diaphragm muscle and breathe more deeply, but not strained. Gradually you will feel an improvement and it will become natural to breathe fully. If you study infants or 'toddlers', you

will see that they have both good postural and breathing habits. Somehow, sadly, most of them will gradually develop bad habits as they get older. Taking in sufficient quantities of oxygen is important in the Eight Strands. Follow the advice on breathing with the instructions for each exercise.

The First Qigong Technique.
One thing you can not do and do not want to do is rush your entrance into Qigong. After checking and establishing all your preparations, make your time for regular practice. The first technique is to make contact with your Qi, so to speak. You already have Qi, you just need to become aware of it. Before doing anything, take stock of how you feel, mentally and physically.

Follow this simple check list:
- How does your mind feel, dull, hyperactive, quiet, passive, active, alert?
- How do your hands feel; e.g. cold, not much sensation, hot, clammy?
- How does your body feel inside?
- How do your legs and feet feel?

Use one of the three basic postures which suits you best. Lie, sit or stand quietly. Become aware of your breathing and go through your 'wave' breathing; the diaphragmatic 'Full Breath'.

After your full breathing practice it is time to become aware of your Qi. Run through the above check list again and note any differences. Write them down if you like as a record for later.

Feelings and 'Odd Things'.
It is not uncommon for beginners to experience things that they are not familiar with. This can be misleading or confusing, like learning to use a computer system from scratch is. When we are not used to something we may tend to be unsure whether we are doing the right thing, or in this case "feeling" the right thing. You may experience twitches, itches, tingles, hot or cold sensations on different parts of the limbs, sneezing, small

muscle spasms, "crawling" sensations or a tingling sensation; this can feel like what is commonly called 'pins and needles' that you get when blood circulation has been restricted near nerve endings, but unlike this the tingling sensations move along a limb or over the body across a larger area.

Becoming aware of your Qi, or at least trying to, is a most important part of introductory practice. Most people in this world are far too busy working, travelling or being involved with family and friends to take time out, stop, listen, feel and be aware of themselves in any depth. Therefore most people will miss these ordinary and natural sensations and indeed may find them 'strange' at first, possibly even denying them. Persevere, let your mind rest and leave the daily mayhem behind. Mental 'chatter' is another problem. Every time you try to concentrate on one thing or empty your mind there may be a million seemingly unconnected thoughts swimming frantically around your brain. This can be overcome, with practice. The results are rewarding, as well as surprising.

Practice the combination of the posture, breathing and awareness, until you become settled. This alone is therapeutic and noticeable in its effect on your daily life, so imagine what the fully accomplished exercising will be like.

Second Technique.
Eight Qi Gathering Breaths.

After practising the first technique for at least eight sessions, use your same practice space and time to try the second technique. Circulation of the breath and Qi is a very important step and you will see why I recommend following the 'First Technique' before tackling it, as you are training the mind to focus internally and getting comfortable with posture holding externally, so as to lessen the risk of concentration loss and ensuing disappointment.

Begin by standing in the upright posture, then shift your weight to your right leg. Move the left foot out so the distance between the feet is just over shoulder width. Transfer fifty percent of the weight to the left foot. Bend your knees, as though riding on horse-back. Tuck the pelvis down and forward slightly, so as to straighten the lower spine and keep your head raised aloft, as though being suspended by the Bahui point; between the two actions of raising the head and sinking the pelvis, the spine is kept straight. Relax.

The object of the 'Eight Qi Gathering Breaths' is threefold. Firstly the arm raising movements open up the rib cage and allow the lungs to work to maximum capacity unimpeded. Secondly, the exercise helps train the mind to follow or direct the body's Qi. Thirdly, but not least, it helps build up the strength of the qi, making it ideal as an energy building routine when extra strength and concentration is needed quickly.

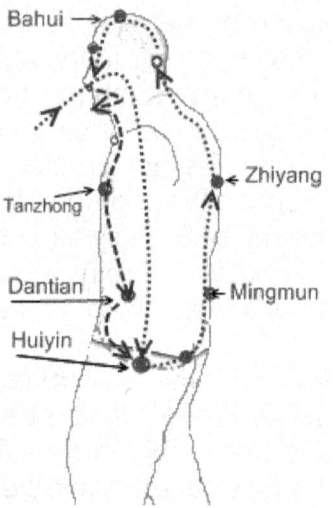

Look at the diagram opposite. Although this diagram is for demonstrating the Microcosmic Orbit, it also serves for illustrating the 'Eight Qi Gathering Breaths' as they are very similar in movement and direction; the main difference being that in Eight Qi Gathering Breaths one does not hold or circulate the Qi at individual points as it is more of a "Qi washing" programme. An advanced version of this exercise takes in the Greater Orbit, heel breathing and combined circulation. This should only be learned after at least six months of building up the main centres and gates.

On the next page you will find illustrations of the 'Eight Qi Gathering Breaths'. Obviously line drawings do not give indication of flow or pressure, tension or relaxation. The body should be as relaxed as possible, especially the shoulders, back and waist. The movements are natural, like combing your hair or getting dressed. Let each circulation of Qi be in time with the breathing; you may experience a slight slowing down as you go from the first to the eighth, that is natural and is called "settling". Focus on the exercise.

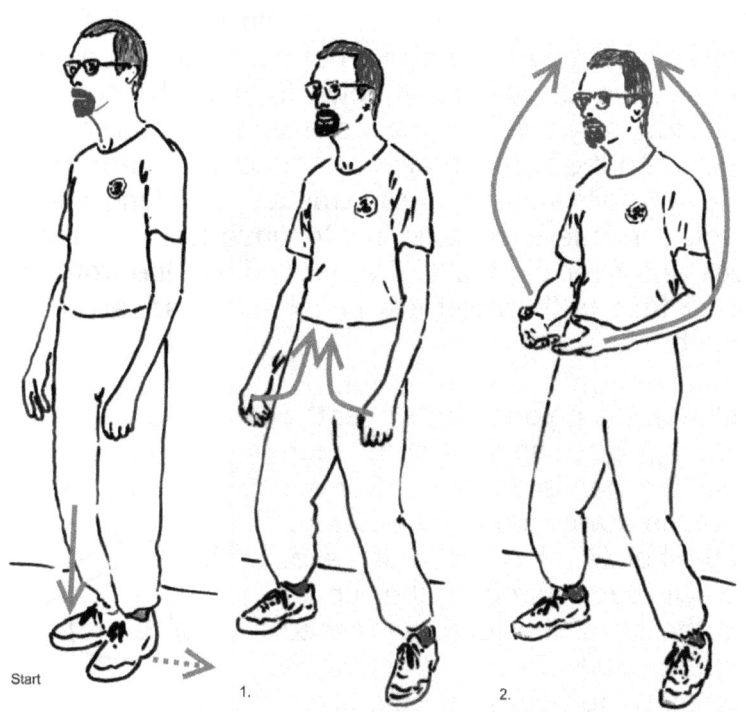

Begin from 'Eagle Stance' (feet together at the heels, knees slightly bent, arms by sides) and clear your mind – Illustration labelled 'Start', above top left. Drop the weight down onto the right leg and step out to shoulder's width apart with the right foot. This is called 'Horse Riding Stance or Ma bu (1.). From the Horse-riding Stance, exhale to clear the lungs of stale air and gasses. Bring both hands down to the sides, turning the palms forwards, as though preparing to lift something (2.). Next, in a smooth and continuous movement, you inhale, raise both arms, palms up and open, as though lifting a large beach ball up to head level (3.); do this without putting tension into the shoulders, arching your back or raising your height by straightening the legs. As you inhale in this action, imagine the Qi coming in with the breath through the top of the head and in through the nose to the

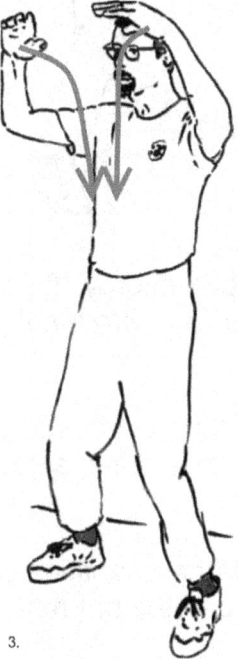

lungs. That Qi, Universal Energy, is coming in with it (dotted line in diagram p.114). As the stream of air reaches the lungs and dissipates, the Qi carries on down through the centre of the torso to the very base of the body and the Huiyin point (situated between the anus and the reproductive organ). Using your mind's eye, follow the Qi backwards and up alongside the spine as you continue to breathe in. Continue to follow the Qi up the neck and over the top of the head, down the front and middle of the face to the point just below the nose, all on the slow in-breath.

Exhaling slowly, bring your hands over the head, as though washing your head, then slowly lower the hands down the front of the body, palms downwards and fingertips facing each other (4.). In your mind's eye, follow the Qi back through the upper gums, into the tip of the tongue (dashed line in diagram), down through the tongue to the 'root' of it, then out along the lower palette, through the lower gums and out to a point roughly half-way between the lips and the chin.

The Qi flows down the centre of the chest, stomach and abdomen to the Dantian. Here the 'fresh' Qi is stored, a bit like charging up a battery. Advanced or competent practitioners can imagine that as the 'new Qi' travels down to the Dantian, the 'stale Qi', along with any negative energy, flows down the front of the legs, over the toes and down through the floor via the foot's 'Wellspring Point'.

Repeat this action eight times. Practice this before breakfast, before lunch, and last thing at night before bed. After a few days you should start to notice the effect.

Warning: You may not be used to taking in large quantities of oxygen. If you feel dizzy, stop. Take deeper breaths but never strain or force it. The whole process should become natural after a few dozen practice sessions.

Important Notes:
Start in your preferred posture. Firstly practice mindfulness and diaphragmatic breathing (a.k.a. Dantian Breathing). After a few breaths, relax. Now as you lie/sit/stand, follow the breath in through your nose, down the windpipe and into the lungs. The breath dissipates through the lungs and around the blood circulatory system.

Bear in mind that the tongue is lightly turned upwards, the tip connecting to the upper palette or roof of the mouth, acting like a switch on the central meridians and connecting the Governor Vessel (back) with the Conception Vessel (front).

In Tiandidao Kuoshu (Traditional Chinese Arts, the Way of Heaven & Earth), this exercise is used as a prelude for training and can also be used as a Qi centring method at the end of sessions. All students of Qigong (including Baduanjin), Taijiquan and Dowist Gongfu are taught this exercise as a prelude to training as well as being a quick 'energiser' and 'leveller'.

Third Technique.
Expanding the Dantian

Also known in another context as 'Qi Centring', this exercise is more concerned with the mindfulness and wilful direction of Qi, an important aspect of training. There are many variations of exercise in which the practitioner uses concentration – Mind's Will ('I' pronounced "Yee" in Chinese), most doing the same thing, getting the practitioner to feel and take control of their own Qi. This one is included here because it is an important aspect of not only basic Qigong for health but Martial Qigong too: in all forms of Internal Kung Fu the practitioner begins by centring their Qi at the lower Dantian before commencing Form; in Taijiquan this is usually referred to as 'Attaining Wuji', a different slant but nevertheless the same method used to different ends.

In Qigong for health you need to learn to centre the Qi at the abdominal Dantian before circulating it around the body as a 'washing' or 'strengthening' force. Many of the original Chinese concepts and instructions can be very confusing, even misleading, about this aspect. Translation from Chinese to English can be very ambiguous at the best of times, but added to this is many people's individual translation based upon (a) their knowledge of both languages, and (b) their knowledge of the methods, broad scale or narrow. Such difficulties have led to many misunderstandings. One of these is 'centring' and what you are actually doing. This needs to be explained in great detail, so as the practitioner, especially the novice, is clear about what he or she is trying to achieve before setting out.

Definitions:
1. In health practice the Qi is 'centred' at the Dantian to help increase mindfulness, build up power and to regulate the Qi as well as gather it; as many untrained people's Qi may be 'scattered' or irregular. This is linked to medical ideology but of the most important and typically Chinese idea of self-help, Preventative Medicine. To use another one of my famous analogies, this is a bit like looking after your car, keeping electrical circuits clean and working effectively. In the case of building up Qi at the lower Dantian it is like charging the battery, where reserve power is also kept, but it is still charged up every time you use the vehicle (exercise). To start your "vehicle" every day you need power, this turns over the electric starting motor, powers the spark plugs and gets you going. Qigong for health is like car maintenance, the more you look after it, the less it will let you down.

2. In Martial Qigong, as mentioned above, the Qi is centred at the abdominal Dantian prior to any action or movement. This is also linked to having a quiet Mind –

empty. An analogy I use for this is the heart of your Personal Computer (PC), the Central Processor Unit (CPU) or 'Chip'. This vital piece of processing power is the brain of the computer. To use it it needs to be empty, then information can be put into it from whence the CPU processes it and passes it out as an action or command. If the CPU did not pass the information through but held everything in Memory without action, it becomes "full" and can not continue to process. We usually associate this with a 'crash' and a "blue window of death", very familiar to most PC users! If we are confronted with a personal emergency, like self-defence, and the mind is filled with more things than the brain can process, then panic sets in and we 'freeze', just like the computer. Learning to centre the Qi and empty the mind increases processing power so that this "emergency information" can be passed through as quickly as possible and "actioned"; used for response. This response is formed via training in movements, Kung Fu (Trained Skills), all designed to meet different physical situations.

Hopefully the two basic definitions above will help clear your mind about what you are trying to achieve as well as eliminate any misconceptions previously learned. In the following exercise you will be taken through the simple, yet demanding process of concentrating your Qi at the Dantian. One more thing we should make clear about this is that we are not stopping the Qi, allowing it to stagnate, nor are we stopping the flow of Qi in any of the Meridians (energy channels). As long as Qi flows there is life. When you concentrate on the Dantian you are building up the strength of your personal Qi, like charging a battery, and centring any excess Qi, thereby regulating it. This exercise leads on to other training methods whereby you can concentrate and guide the Qi around smaller energy points, or 'gates', as illustrated in the fourth technique, Microcosmic Orbit: do not skip this section as you will get better results.

Expanding the Dantian.

Method:
Begin with the usual preparations. Get comfortable and make sure that you will not be disturbed. For the illustration here I have used the seated posture, this may be preferable to most people, especially if they find standing uncomfortable and therefore distracting. Keep the spine erect, neither leaning forwards, backwards nor slumping (curved).

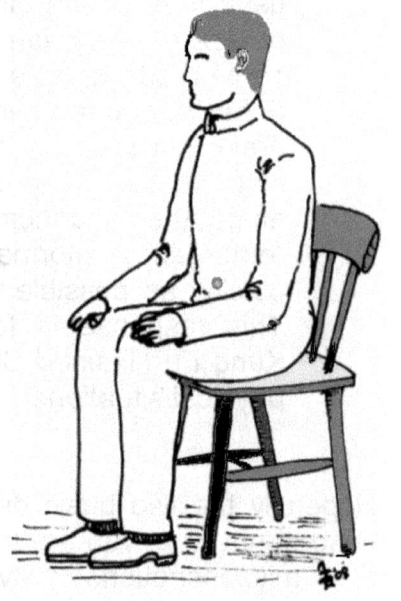

Start your relaxed but deep breathing. This should be focussed upon until you achieve a regular breathing pattern. Your eyes, in the beginning, should always settle on the horizon; imagine that you can see the horizon eight miles away. With your 'mind's-eye' slowly look downwards and inwards until you settle at a point approximately two inches below the Navel and three inches inside the abdominal cavity. In terms of alignment, this point should be directly below the Pineal Gland outlet that we call the 'third eye'.

Imagine the Qi coming into the body with every breath. This can be done in the manner of the Qi gathering breaths exercise, or, quite simply, imagine that the Qi is just pouring into the body as you breathe and filling up the Dantian slowly. If you wish you can imagine this stream of Qi as a coloured 'mist' which can be bright 'electric blue'. For healing purposes it can be bright green, the colour of summer grass.

After a few minutes you should begin to feel a warm sensation in the abdominal area where the Dantian is situated. Allow this to continue: this will only happen if your concentration is strong and uninterrupted. Keep building up the Qi and imagine that your Dantian is getting bigger and stronger. Maintain the session until you begin to grow weary. Always finish with an affirmation such as, "My Qi is getting stronger. My health is getting better."

By practising this exercise two or three times a day in the early stages you will not only strengthen your Qi but also your concentration and resolve. Keep practising, whether or not you feel the warmth building up at the Dantian. On occasions you may feel other sensations, like a cool spot, tingling or even a kind of tickling, like the proverbial butterflies in the stomach.

Support.
On the subject of affirmations again, a really good one is the well known curative of words, "Every day, in every way, I am getting better". Repeat affirmations to yourself until you can say it with conviction. This is a great way of changing your mental state from negative to positive.

At this stage you can also use affirmations as a pre-sleep method of achieving goals, last thing as you close your eyes to sleep. For example, "As I sleep my body will heal and my body become stronger." Or, one that can also be used at any time of the day, "My body is as strong as a mountain. My Mind as clear as a flowing mountain stream." Try some affirmations for yourself, you will find them a very useful accompaniment to Qigong.

Fourth Technique.
Microcosmic Orbit.

Stand, sit or lie in a posture that suits your health status best: standing or sitting will reap the best results.

The diagram right is included again here for your convenience. Next we shall extend this mindfulness of breath to include Qi and some of the main points on the central meridians. These central meridians or channels are considered the main distributory channels and the Governing Vessel contains points which relate to all the main organs and their channels. We are going to circulate the Qi around these channels, briefly concentrating on each of the labelled points as we do so. This has a 'washing' effect and helps clear blockages, strengthen Qi flow and gain mental control over your bioenergies.

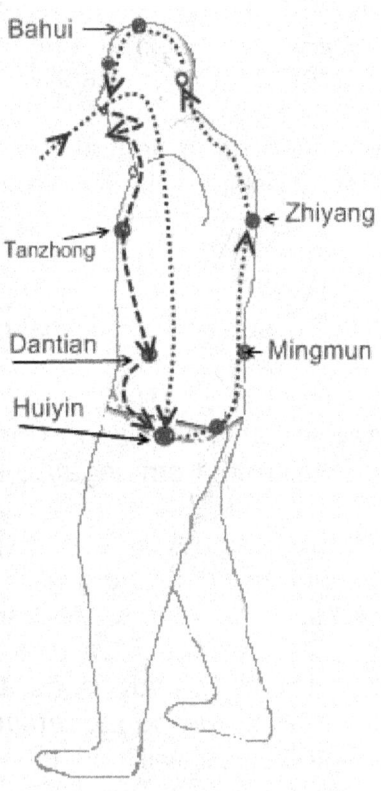

The Microcosmic Orbit

You do not have to move your arms for this exercise, so they can be left by your sides, or on your lap if seated. Imagine that as you draw the breath in through the nose to the lungs that Qi, Universal Energy, is coming in with it (dotted line in diagram). As the stream of air reaches the lungs and dissipates, the Qi carries on down through the centre of the torso to the very base of the body and the Huiyin point (situated between the anus and the reproductive organ). The path the Qi takes then continues up along the path of the spine, and the back of the neck and over the top centre of the head, down the front and middle of the face to the point just below the nose.

From here bear in mind that the tongue is lightly turned upwards, the tip connecting to the upper palette or roof of the mouth, acting like a switch on the central meridians and connecting the Governor Vessel (back) with the Conception Vessel (front). The Qi follows the Conception Vessel (Ren Mai) back through the upper gums, into the tip of the tongue (dashed line in diagram), down through the tongue to the 'root' of it, then out along the lower palette, through the lower gums and out to a point roughly half-way between the lips and the chin.

The Qi flows down the centre of the chest, stomach and abdomen to the groin, then back to the Huiyin point. This is the basic Microcosmic Orbit, utilising the two major energy channels. Synchronising breath, mind and Qi helps 'wash' the channels, improve the Qi flow, unlock 'gates' and stabilise Qi flow as well as improving awareness and mindful Qi guidance. This exercise clears and 'charges' the main gates and points on the central meridians known as (in order from the base point):

- Huiyin – base of body
- Dantian (inner) – centre of abdomen
- Dantian (outer)
- Mingmun – lower back
- Zhiyang - Upper back, between shoulder-blades
- Bahui – Top centre of head (Pineal Gland)
- Xuanguan – 'Third Eye' (Pineal Outlet)
- Tanzhong – Heart Region or Upper Dantian

The Qi also passes through many other points en route, including the Shenting and Renzhong points on the front and Jaiji, Dazhui and Yamen points on the back, which all have a beneficial added effect from this "Qi wash". There is a third channel in theory which travels down the centreline of the body from the Bahui point to the Huiyin point, used in visualisation, but here I have combined this with the in breath, as my Old Master taught. Some people use other exercises to warm-up or prepare for this, like the arm raising exercise; similar to the 'Mexican Wave' performed by football fans, etcetera, but more slowly and combined with breathing in on the upward movement and out on lowering. This is said to "open the energy channels", but quite honestly if your energy channels are not open and functional already you will be in deep trouble... or dead! On a less light-hearted note, the energy channels may be "boosted" before doing the Microcosmic Orbit exercise. This can be done using the Eight Qi Gathering Breaths.

There are two main methods of doing this exercise, as far as I am aware, there may be more. As long as you can get on with one method, it does not really matter which one you choose to perform.

Method One:
Start by gathering the Qi at the Dantian.
At no time should you hold the breath or be tense.
As you breathe in, move Qi from the Dantian to the Huiyin point and hold it at that point for eight seconds. Exhale after counting eight. On the next inhalation, move the Qi from the Huiyin point to the Mingmun point, lower back, and again hold the Qi there for eight seconds. Exhale. Inhale, move the Qi up to the Zhiyang point between the lower aspect of the Shoulder-blades. On the next inhalation, move the Qi to the Bahui point and hold. Follow on to the Xuanguan point, holding the Qi for eight seconds. Next move on to the point where the two central meridians meet, below the nose, just above the upper lip. With the tongue touching the upper palate, the connection is made from Governing Vessel to Conception Vessel and the Qi can flow down through the upper palate, through the tongue to the 'root', out through the lower palate and to a point between the lower lip and chin – central. The next point to hold the Qi at for eight seconds is the Tanzhong, or Heart-level Dantian. Lastly centre the Qi at the Dantian.

Method Two:
Start by gathering the Qi at the Dantian.
At no time should you hold the breath or be tense.
As you breathe in, move Qi from the Dantian to the Huiyin point and with your Mind's eye follow the Qi around all the points. As it reaches each point visualise the Qi 'washing' around each point before moving on to the next. Some people

may find it easier to visualise the Qi washing around each point on the in breath, then moving on to the next point whilst breathing out and thereby keeping an even flow of mind, Qi and breath.

Different teachers teach different ways but it is the point of the exercise which is most important, not so much the method. The point of this qigong exercise, like so many, is to clear the 'gates', strengthen the flow of Qi and thereby improve the health.

Moving Qi.
There are many Qigong exercises which are designed to familiarise the new student of Qigong with using the mind to move Qi around the body. What you have to realise is that these are all a matter of personal preference or different styles of teaching. For example, you may consider gathering the Qi at the Dantian, then 'washing' the Qi down the left arm as you exhale, then bring it back up again, taking it back to the Dantian, via the armpit, as you inhale. Then do the same with the right arm. After this you can circulate or wash the Qi down the right then left legs, each time centring at the Dantian upon the 'return'. This aids concentration and at the same time improves Qi flow.

Other exercises of this nature can include circulating Qi from the P9 point (hand Laogong) to the fingertips and back. There are also many which concentrate on specifics, like clearing the head, but these should only be attempted under close instruction from a qualified teacher.

In Martial Qigong the Qi is not only moved within one's own body but also transmitted to an opponent, this can be done in different ways to achieve different results. As I do not advocate the open teaching of this subject and think that it would be irresponsible, this is not the place to go any further with the subject of Martial Qigong.

Healing Qigong also uses transmitted Qi, from the "healer" to the "patient", a familiar occurrence in China. It is also familiar in lesser degrees in the West as a formalised Qigong balancing method is frequently found here, Reiki Therapy. Reiki was, like so many Japanese Arts, imported over from China. Some enterprising person had the idea to formalise it and also ritualise it, then passing it on to others. Reiki begins with a ceremonious opening of the energy channels for the 'initiate'. Usually the initiate has to sit quietly with his or her eyes closed, so this 'secret' is not passed on too easily.

The basic idea of Healing Qigong is that the person who transmits his or her Qi to another 'channels' the energies of the Universe, or World, "Weiqi" to the recipient's main energy centres - as detailed above. This "charges" the recipient's energy system and helps them achieve balance, where balance was lost.

There are many traditional Chinese methods of Qi emitting, using either mind and a static posture or a gently moving method where Qi is directed; usually at closer ranges. Using the static posture, like a meditation pose, Qi can be transmitted over distances, sometimes great distances. In my experience there has to be some sort of connection between the recipient and the transmitter. In traditional qigong, many practising Masters agree that this connection should at least be a mutually arranged time with "mental" connecting. Of course, sceptics may argue that if such an arrangement was made with prearranged time schedules, then it could be that the recipient is being tricked by their own mind into thinking that something is happening. Let the sceptics remain ignorant, I say, until something positive happens to them to perhaps persuade themselves that the opposite is in fact true. There again, perhaps they prefer to remain sceptic as they may be frightened of the "unknown" and unseen forces in life; psychology is an interesting subject! Experiencing Qi projection to another person has been one of my personal achievements; around 1997-8 one of my female students telephoned me to ask about something, and during the conversation made an "ow!" noise. I asked was she all right and she replied that due to Period Pain she had a very uncomfortable pain in her abdominal area. With no hint as to what I was doing I immediately carried on a normal conversation but consciously expressed Qi to her. After a few moments she giggled and said, "Mike, what are you doing?", "Why?" was my reply. "Well, where I had that pain a minute ago it's now tingling, like a tickling sensation and it feels much better. Is it you.... are you giving me your Qi?", she asked. "Yes. Glad to be of help!" Trish lived on the opposite side of the city to me, so was about four miles away. As mentioned elsewhere in this book, Qi is just like other energy transmissions, like television, radio or Morse code, so if you believe in television you might as well accept Qi transmission too.

Shih-fu Soo not only mentioned this to us in his classes, he used it, frequently! His Qi emissions were strong and could not only be felt but could sometimes be seen too; like when he passed his Qi through a tumbler of water in a darkened room. Shih-fu Wong, Kiew Kit, also talks about Qi transmission in his wonderful book 'Qigong for Health and Vitality', which came to my attention just a few years after studying with Shih-fu Soo, being at a time when there were many ignorant people (who had never even practised Qigong!) saying that such things were impossible and could not exist. Having personally experienced the power of Qi transmission, both on the above occasion and others, it was no surprise to me, but when I think of how Shih-fu Soo must have suffered in silence over the doubters and name callers is very upsetting to me, one of his most admiring students who is also very grateful for his openness in teaching and sharing his profound knowledge and his unswerving dedication to his students.

Heaven and Earth Qigong.
An advanced exercise in Tiandidao school is 'Tiandi Qigong', or Heaven and Earth Energy Training. This exercise is not fully illustrated or written herein. In this method the practitioner uses a tree for strengthening Weiqi Qigong practice. By using this method in advanced stage, he or she develops far greater ability to transmit or receive Qi over distances. Again the instructor's guidance and watchful eye is essential.

Qigong Walking.
Another simple yet effective Qigong exercise is a walking method that anyone who can walk can do. It has renowned effects on many common illnesses, including cancers, lung disease and heart problems: for example, someone who has had a heart attack but is still able to walk, may benefit from doing this exercise slowly with the coordinated breathing. A person with severe respiratory disease, such as Tuberculosis, may benefit from a more brisk walk to help strengthen and replenish the lungs and bronchial tubes. This has been used in TCM for many years now and has helped thousands of people.

Method:
Begin from an even stance such as Eagle Stance or Bear Stance – feet beside each other, weight distributed evenly. The body should be upright but relaxed, as is common for almost all Qigong and Taijiquan. It is important to keep the shoulders relaxed, even when moving.
1. Transfer the weight to the right foot and leg; keep the knee 'soft' or bent for balance.
2. When the left leg is "empty" of weight, place the left foot outwards and forwards slightly resting it on the heel. Allow both your arms to swing forwards and leftwards at the same time, palms upwards - as though about to receive a tray. Breathe in as you do this step and arm swing.
3. As you inhale and transfer all the weight to the left leg, culminating the full breath with the end of the weight transference, sink and relax the waist and shoulders, but without slumping. With all the weight now on the left foot...
4. ... extend the right "empty" foot forwards and slightly outwards. As you begin to transfer the weight to the right leg and foot, exhale naturally and swing both arms rightwards across the body as though receiving a tray.
5. Continue this method of stepping for as long as possible; slowly for those who have suffered heart problems or strokes, but faster for those who have had lung problems or are overweight.

Obviously, due to the nature of the arm swinging, you will need a wide enough space to practice this walk so a hallway or alleyway may not suffice. A park or garden would be fine, but in western society many people may feel self-conscious doing this exercise by itself, so doing it in a private garden might be preferred. In the early 1990's I used to stop in the Chapelfield Gardens (public park) on my way back from the city shops to do some Qigong and Taijiquan. At first I thought I might get passing youths making childish comments, or people asking questions, but not a soul appeared to pay the slightest bit of attention. Try going to your local park and see for yourself, nowadays more people are aware of Qigong, or at least Taijiquan, so you may be pleasantly surprised. Better still if you can practice in a class situation, or at least with a friend.

As this is such a simple exercise, once you have got the coordinated stepping and breathing, it is something that can be done whilst walking in the countryside, perhaps along one of the many disused railway tracks that have now been converted to walkways, or any fairly even footpath.

Medical Professionals.

Anyone working within a branch of the medical profession which deals with rehabilitation could try this simple Qigong method under strictly controlled tests: one group suffering the same problems tries the exercise for six months whilst a similar group does not. This type of experiment has been carried out all over the world with Qigong and Dr. Paul Lam's 'Tai Chi for Arthritis', etcetera, all with very pleasing results. To find an instructor of Qigong in your area you can see the list of qualified Tiandidao instructors towards the back of this book or conduct your own search.

Qigong Street Walking.

The above exercise can be discreetly adapted for practice when walking along any street without anyone suspecting that you are doing an exercise regime! Simply follow the same principles, that is to inhale as you step forwards with your left foot and exhale as you step with the right foot. Let the arms swing naturally and concentrate on the breath and step co-ordination instead. This is not quite as beneficial as the complete Qigong Walking exercise but will still have benefits.

Qigong Cycling.

Yes, you read it correctly. You can do the very same exercise whilst cycling as a general Qigong strengthener and exercise. The first priority here is to make sure that the equipment you are using, your bicycle, is the right size for you and that your knees remain bent at the furthest downward stroke of the pedals, your back is reasonably upright and straight: the old style 'upright' bicycle, affectionately known as a "sit up and beg" model, is ideal for posture and control. The most important thing is that you pay attention to the other road users around you! Do not do it in busy areas.

Using the same breathing pattern as Qigong Walking, exhale as you push the left pedal down and inhale as you push the right pedal down. Once this becomes habitual and you do not have to concentrate on breath coordination (please remain safe and concentrate on the road and traffic!), try visualising the Qi washing from the Dantian down to the Yongquan or foot wellspring point as you push each foot downwards, thus washing or pumping Qi through the leg channels. This only needs to be done around sixteen times each side, thirty-two maximum. Obviously the main consideration here is safety: if you lack good road sense or concentration then do not attempt this exercise on a public highway. It is not my intention or the intention of this book to encourage any activity which could lead to injury, of yourself or others, so this exercise is not recommended but only mentioned here out of interest as it may be practised on a cycling exercise machine in the safety of your own home.

Other Qigong Exercises

As mentioned before, there are many qigong exercises, for health, medical application and Martial Arts. Here are just a few of the exercises that we use in Tiandidao Academy.

Opening the Energy Channels.
This is an exercise that should be learned under supervision by an experienced instructor with whom you can communicate about any feelings or changes occurring.

1. Breathe in, draw the Qi from the Dantian down to the Huiyin point, then up the spine and neck to the top of the head – Bahui. Let the Qi settle with your concentration at the Bahui point.
2. Exhale gently as you lower the Qi over the top of the head, down the middle of the face to the upper palate point, through the tongue to the 'root', out through the lower palate and down the centre-front of the body, past the Dantian and back down to the Huiyin.
3. Breathe in and raise the Qi up the front to Dantian height and let it 'split' around the Belt Channel joining up at the Mingmun point at waist level, then along the spine up to the neck area – upper back. Let the Qi settle with the concentration there.
4. Breathe out slowly as you let the Qi 'split' across the back of both shoulders, down the outside of both arms and over the middle fingers, bringing it to the inside palm – P9 point.
5. Inhale and raise the Qi up from the centre of the palms, up the inside arms to the armpits, then down to the points behind the nipples, where again you halt for a second.
6. Breathe out and visualise the Qi travelling downwards to the Belt Channel, then inwards towards the centre and down again towards the genital region and the Huiyin.
7. Inhaling raise the Qi up the centreline to the Upper Dantian or Solar Plexus region – approximately two

inches below heart level – on no account bring the Qi any higher than this.

8. Exhale and sink the Qi downwards again towards the groin where it divides along the outsides of the legs, down to the toes where it goes over the tips and underneath, stopping at the foot wellspring point Yongquan – in the hollow, just behind the ball-of-foot.
9. Breathe in and raise the Qi back over the heels and up the inside of the ankles, legs and groin up to the abdominal Dantian where it settles briefly again.
10. Exhale and allow the Qi to sink to the Huiyin point again, this time allowing it to settle and remain; after having done your repetitions you should concentrate on settling the Qi there whilst your breathing returns to 'normal', do not hold your breath.

Remember the instructions above. It is most important that you are both mentally and physically prepared, and comfortable, before beginning. Qigong is like any other worthwhile endeavour, the better you prepare, the better the results. Also pay heed to the health warnings outlined in an earlier chapter.

Opening the Energy Channels can have very strong effects and some side-effects may be unsettling if the practitioner is of a sensitive nature or prone to worrying. This is why you need a well experienced instructor who is aware of and knows how to deal with these things. Generally speaking, most side-effects are quite mild and nothing at all to worry about, however, humans being humans we vary in strengths and weaknesses, so some may be alarmed where others may barely notice. One of the most common effects is usually described as 'hallucination', but is not what it seems. Practising Qigong, or any other exercise involving deep breathing, can cause changes in blood pressure and this can have an effect on the eyeballs and therefore vision. Nothing to be alarmed by.

Opening the Energy Channels should not be used as a first exercise for those who are ill or weak. As mentioned earlier in this book, exercises like "concentrate on the Dantian" should be done first by those who are ill, weak or overweight. This is another reason why the unenlightened should never attempt to learn from books or videos; these mediums are fine for extra aid in learning from a competent instructor though, but only as a reminder of detail, aide de memoir.

The Roaming Heavenly Dragon.

It was not until the 1950's that the meditative, healing and corrective skills of using the breath became known as 'Qigong'. Each method (Fa) employed was just an exercise which bore a name that related, usually, to its main character. Some of these names seem quite strange to westerners, like 'Tortoise Breathing', 'Heel Breathing', 'Focusing One' or 'Eating Six Energies' for example. To the inquisitive and probing Chinese Mind these are very apt names. Tortoise Breathing uses the nostrils to control the flow of breath combined with some physical posturing and mindfulness. This simply comes from observing a Tortoise and how it breathes using its nostrils to control airflow. Taoists believed that partially due to this method of breathing the Tortoise owed its long life, so set about copying it and observing results. They also believed that there are six main energies within the Universe, so 'eating' these energies or absorbing them thoroughly would be good for the practitioner.

What of the Dragon? We know that in reality Dragons do not exist, but in the mind and hearts of the Chinese people they do. There are many kinds of Dragons, as discussed earlier, but the Heavenly Dragon is perhaps one of the most revered. The roofs of traditional Chinese buildings, like Temples, have "turned up" corners to them and slope down less at the edges. This is so that the Heavenly dragons may sleep on the roof tops at night without falling off. This respect for the spirit is not only amusing but quite charming too, respectful of that which can not be seen as well as that which can.

The Heavenly Dragon roams the sky and it is this concept that the exercise uses as a visualisation for the practitioner. Visualisation is very important in all forms of Qigong for it is the Mind which controls the will to guide the Qi; this is called Mind's Intent, or Hsing-I ("Xingyi", with the 'X' pronounced like "Xz" as in Zone) in Chinese. In Chinese Boxing (nick-named

Kung Fu) there are many styles which mimic animals, such as Tiger, Crane, Monkey and Snake; Dragon is meant to be a kind of accumulation of other animal styles, representative of 'Spirit' (Shen). In Heavenly Dragon, as with all animal styles, it is essential for the practitioner to visualise being that animal. The Dragon, as artistically reproduced, has the head of a cat, the body of a snake, the claws of a cat and is enhanced with supernatural powers and properties. Visualisation of this when performing the exercise will help get the best results. Be a Dragon roaming the Heavens!

Characteristics of this exercise are:
1. Use Dragon Claws, stretched and relaxed[6].
2. Begin with Dragon Awakes; stretching, yawning, etc.
3. Use Dragon Stances sometimes (similar to Bow Stance or Gong Bu), as well as crouching, swooping, flying and pausing or stopping (like a cat).
4. Let the body move like a snake, a stealthy cat and a lizard, making spontaneous twists, turns, leaning and other actions like the combined animals.
5. Imagine that you are searching amongst the clouds, therefore sometimes parting clouds with your claws, looking, playing, examining and moving on.
6. Allow all movements to be spontaneous and free, do not think twice or block the natural flow. Therefore, if you suddenly feel like doing a little wiggle, scratching your head, shaking your tail or yawning, just do it - this is just your body telling you what it needs to do!
7. Allow natural breathing at all times, do not even think about breathing.
8. Let the exercise take as long as it takes, you will know when it is time to finish as your body will tell you.

As you can ascertain from the above list, this is an exercise where body and consciousness communicate and you act in accordance with their need. This way the body can 'direct you', so to speak, and correct any imbalances, stiff joints, out of tune Meridians and so on. In fact, all that is really happening is that for once you are switching off from the outside world and

---

[6]For information on Dragon Claw and Stance work, see the book, 'Kung Fu – The Way of Heaven and Earth', available from all booksellers.

"listening" to your body and energies and letting them communicate their needs through your conscious pursuit of this method. Hence, when the work is done you will "feel" it and be conscious of the fact that it is time to stop. With regular practice you will be equally conscious of when it is time to do the exercise; which conjures up wonderful images of someone in a large office building, suddenly getting up from their desk and becoming a Heavenly Dragon!

The Heavenly Roaming Dragon is a wonderful exercise to teach children as they are, or at least should be, more adept at using their imagination. One of my past Taoist Yoga trainees was a Primary School Teacher and she did it in a free period with her group of children. She reported that they thoroughly enjoyed it and were bright eyed, attentive and in a good mood for the rest of the day. Children are rarely taught any worthwhile exercises at school in the Western Hemisphere, so what a brilliant way to get children to get in touch with their bodies, minds and physical well-being. Exercise with multi-purpose.

Lifting The Sky.
This Qigong method is beneficial to all whether a Master or Novice. To perform it is very simple yet the results are positive and health enhancing. Although the movements are easy to do it is not the physical aspect which you should concentrate on. The main aim is to feel the energy flow. Physically, as is the case for all Internal Method (Nei Fa) Qigong, you should be relaxed. Your breathing should be deep but natural, never force the breath or breathe loudly, keeping it quiet and calm. Likewise your Mind should be quiet and calm, not letting your thoughts wander.

Method:
1. Stand upright with your feet about shoulders' width apart (Bear Stance). Let your shoulders relax, knees 'soft', arms hanging by sides with palms facing legs, fingertips naturally relaxed and curved.

2. Exhale. Bring your hands up to Dantian level, palms facing up and fingertips pointing towards each other – as illustrated to the right. At this point your eyes should be gazing at the horizon, your Qi centred at the Dantian.
3. Breathe in as you turn the palms over and slowly raise them in an outward arc (image two, right) until they are above your head, palms upwards and elbows still curved, so forming a large arc shape above your head. As the hands pass eye level allow the eyes to follow them up, looking between the two hands.
4. On reaching the apex, without strain, hold your breath and push both hands upwards as though raising the sky in a gentle stretching movement.
5. Release the stretch and begin to lower the arms in a large outward (to sides) arcing movement, as though describing a huge circle, outwards and down towards the sides of the hips. Inhale for the first third of the movement, then exhale through the mouth for the last two-thirds, from shoulder height downwards. As you lower the hands, return the eyes to horizon. Feel the Qi flowing down over the head, neck and shoulders then washing down over the body as you lower the arms.
6. Repeat 8, 16 or 24 times in all.

Below is an exercise which looks similar but is completely different in both movement and effects. Both exercises have strong curative values and health enhancing properties whilst being at the same time a 'specific' medical qigong exercise which may be prescribed by a physician for particular illnesses. Whilst these may be taught and learned in a class or seminar my recommendation would be to learn them and only use them infrequently or when needed. If you are an experienced instructor, whilst being acceptive to your Teacher's way and of course respectful, then you decide, based on knowledge common sense never follow blindly.

Carrying the Moon.

Said to "invoke youthfulness", this exercise is highly acclaimed by Qigong Masters and practitioners. With regular practice it is said to make you feel younger and live longer. No ordinary exercise enjoys this kind of eulogy, so given the many good reports this Qigong classic must be doing something right. This exercise requires a deep stretch of the back and preferably locking out the knees, stretching the backs of the legs and the spine dramatically; hence reasonable flexibility is necessary.

Method:
1. Stand upright and relaxed, feet close together but not touching.
2. Allow your back to relax as you slowly 'droop' your body forwards, exhaling, and allow your arms to flop down naturally. On the full bend you should allow your knees to lock out, eyes gazing back through the legs. Feel the Qi running down along the spine, from the Huiyin point at the base, to the Bahui point at the top of the head.
3. Straighten up slowly as you breathe in. Keep your arms straight but not tense, so that they are raised in front of the body. Raise the arms above the head as you straighten into the fully upright position. Bend the elbows outwards so that the shape the arms make above your head is like that of a full, round moon. Also form a moon shape with the thumbs and fingers – as though holding a ball. Continue the upwards stretch until you lean backwards slightly, being careful not to compress the spine. Carry the moon just behind and above your head. Hold the posture and your breath for a count of two.
4. Straighten your body and begin to lower your arms to your sides as you slowly exhale through your mouth. At the same time, visualise the Qi flowing down from your head, cascading like water down the length of the whole body, right down to the fingertips and toes.
5. When you are upright, hands hanging naturally by your sides, stand quietly and relaxed. Enjoy the feeling of the Qi refreshing your body and nourishing every cell as it also eliminates negative waste: think of the cascading

Qi eliminating illness, imbalances and negative emotions being washed out through the soles of the feet.
6. Repeat the exercise eight to ten times, increase to sixteen and later twenty as you begin to feel more fit and younger.

Please remember that today's society is far different from olden days, even just fifty years ago in rural areas. People are used to a more "comfortable" lifestyle, sitting on padded chairs that give you badly stretched or strained back muscles, stooped over computers, driving too much and walking too little, and so on. Obviously I put the word comfortable in parenthesis because it is for the most part a complete misnomer, a fallacy even. Back problems are very common nowadays so it is essential that the would be practitioner of exercises such as Carrying The Moon work on getting their general fitness levels to acceptable standards before attempting anything which utilises the back muscles so much.

This exercise certainly has a very pronounced effect. One thing which is quite clearly felt is the flow of blood as you bend and straighten. This should not be allowed to confuse or distract the practitioner who should concentrate on Qi flow; distinctly different to blood flow. Good concentration is a must, so perhaps the discerning instructor will choose as a prelude some exercising which has more of a meditation value; to meditate is to concentrate on one thing.

Dynamic Qigong.
The Qigong methods described in this book comprise around 75% – 80% of the 'Soft Style' Qigong found in Tiandidao Academy. All of the exercises described above are 'soft' or 'Yin' Qigong because they do not use any muscular tension or forced breathing. As mentioned elsewhere, there is Yin (Internal) Qigong and Yang (External) Qigong, I call Yang Qigong "Dynamic Qigong"; the reason for this being that it shares common traits with Dynamic Tension exercising; muscle toning and building without equipment. Most External or Dynamic Qigong is associated with Martial Arts training, such as Shaolin Quan. However, this association is not correct

by itself as Dynamic Qigong is also used in some Taoist styles as well as in general health and fitness training. As a method of building physical strength it ranks far more highly than weight training, "free weights" that is, as using fixed equipment is even less beneficial; the body was not born and did not grow by being fixed to a frame which limited movement, it develops through free movement, so in that reckoning free weights are better than fixed weights at least, but dynamic muscle and ligament use is even more beneficial as it gives us a more wholesome use of muscle, ligament and connective tissue.

How does it work?
There has never, to my knowledge, been an answer to this age old question. Most qigong practitioners just do as they are shown and the Chinese belief in "If it works, use it. If it does not work, forget it!" has its role to play in this aspect to. However, after many years of Qigong practice (I lost count, but it must be over 38 now, including Pranayama, Meditations and other "breathing work") I have studied this and formed a personal theory. There are certain elements that I have experimented with and taken note of over the years and in some areas a consistency of result or action seems to infer that certain elements take place with specific exercises. The theory is as following:

- Dynamic Tension requires concentrating on a group of muscles which apply force against each other; e.g. the push and pull muscles or extend and retract muscles.
- All methods of Qigong use concentration to focus Qi at a specific point or to circulate it in either a small or larger area.
- Internal Qigong uses relaxed muscles and balanced framework so that the Qi can flow freely.
- External Qigong tenses the muscles, restricting the flow of Qi while they are tensed, then releasing a surge of Qi as they are relaxed; the Mind still concentrating the Qi in that region.
- The muscles in their normal state use Qi; as demonstrated when a baby – who's muscles are not yet developed – grips your little finger quite firmly and apparently without effort. A trained Qigong practitioner

or Internal Martial artist can lift a heavy object in an apparently relaxed state, using Qi to assist in framework and muscle function.

Thus external Qigong works by utilising dynamic tensing of the musculature, which does two things: a) builds up muscle and connecting tissue strength and b) thereby increases not only external muscle strength but their capacity to store and use Qi; Qi can be stored in body tissue and each individual cell has an energy store system which uses Mitochondria as part of the body's energy store and transfer system. The practitioner of External Qigong in Martial Arts can train to discharge sudden or seemingly explosive bursts of energy with quick, hard punches or kicks. This is not to say that a practitioner of Internal Qigong Martial Arts could not do the same thing though and this is why some people choose one method, some the other, depending on the advice they get from their teacher and his or her experience.

Examples of External Qigong vary from school to school, system to system, but listed here are just a few from the Tiandidao school used in both the Daoist Gongfu (Taoist Kung Fu), general health Qigong practises and in Taijiquan.

- Pushing Front and Rear (looking back).
- Four Directional Qigong (in Mabu)
- Alternate Arms (similar to Wing Chun's 'Wrist Block' exercises.)
- Qigong with free weights.
- Tearing Heavy Cotton (as a prelude to Tearing Silk.)
- Dynamic Kicking.
- Dynamic Torso.
- Dynamic Taiji Gongfu[7] (using similarities of weighting, Dantian and energy flow.)

An exercise which strengthens the body's external tissues against blows could be added here as it is, strictly speaking, External Qigong, but it uses different principles, so let us categorise it under a general heading of 'Conditioning'.

---

[7]This aspect, Dynamic Taiji Gongfu, is one found in Tiandidao Form practises as part of the "San Gong Fa"

Dynamic Mabu Exercise.

Included here is an exercise from the Dynamic Qigong range which is generally called 'Four Directional Breathing'. This features the use of Mabu or Horse-riding Stance, which is probably the most popular stance in Chinese exercise. Mabu has always been accredited with building strength in the legs and lower back as well as developing strong Qi. This particular exercise is associated with many aspects of Qigong and variations can be found in almost every Taoist and Buddhist school. This one I learned from Shih-fu Soo as part of the Qi building routines.

Beginners would find this very tiring at first, even though it has just two to eight repetitions. It will make the palms sweat profusely as well as making the leg muscles ache. Stay with it and do not be put off by a few aches, just think of the strength you will be gaining over time. Concentrate on the movements and breathing and success will come.

Four Directional Breathing.

Preparation. Only perform this exercise after general warm-up exercises and *before* medical or general health Qigong, giving time for rest and Qi settlement in-between sessions.

1. Stand quietly as you concentrate your Qi at the lower Dantian and focus on the nature and sequence of the exercise.
2. Shift your weight to your right leg and take the left foot out to shoulder's width or slightly wider: Mabu can also be attained by using 'Four Point Horse-riding Method'. Shift the weight to the left leg and take the right foot out a little further – the stance needs to be wide enough to accommodate a deep knee bend. Bring the weight back to 50-50, make sure that the feet are pointing forwards, bend the knees slightly and drop your weight down, but keep the spine erect.
3. Raise your arms so the hands are in front of the armpits. Bend the fingers over and thumbs in and flex the wrists back so that your palms point forwards. Inhale as you do this.

4. Relax the jaw, allowing the lower and upper teeth to be parted. Push both hands forward as you lower slightly in your stance and push using dynamic force, as though trying to push an invisible wall in front of you (1). As you perform this exhale through your mouth – this makes a hissing sound. Completion of push and breath should be coincidental. When finished, relax and breathe in as you bring your hands back to the starting position (as illustrated below).
5. Repeat the push, this time above your shoulders (2). The palms face upwards, as though pushing an invisible ceiling upwards. Again, relax and return to the original posture when this movement is completed.

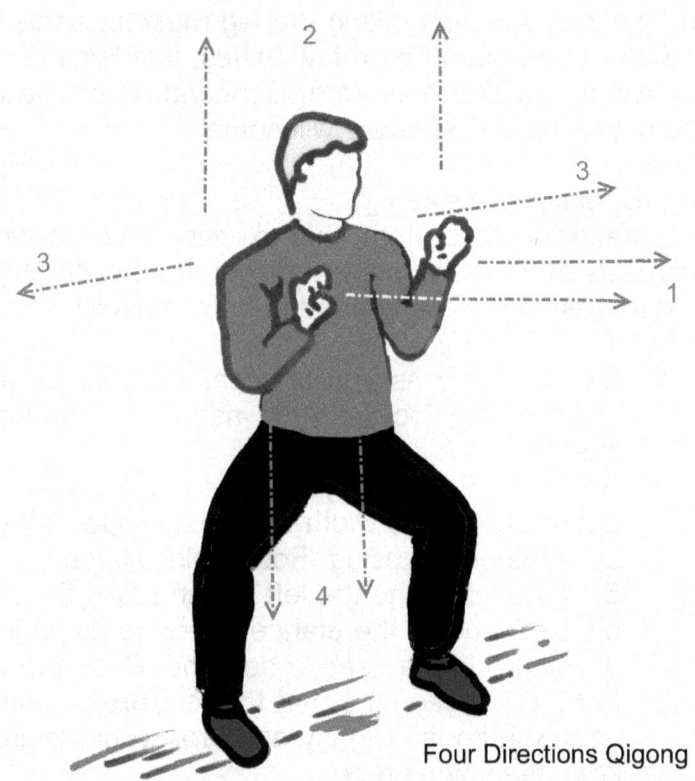

Four Directions Qigong

6. Sequence three (3) is pushing out left and right at the same time, as though trying to push away two walls at your sides. Do not forget to lower your posture as you push in each sequence putting in maximum effort. Relax, inhale and return to the starting posture.

7. The next sequence (4) is downwards. Push both hands, palms facing downwards, between the thighs. As you do this you should bend the legs even further than before, but no more than thighs parallel to the floor. On complete exhalation relax and stand higher again, but do not straighten the legs.
8. Repeat the whole exercise again, all four sequences. You should do this a minimum of two times and a maximum of eight.

Notes: Never do exercises like this and just walk away. In a program of exercises this type is best done around one-third of the way through, for example, so that you finish with "soft style" Qigong, Forms or warm-downs and centring. This all depends on the structure of your system and what your Teacher (Shih-fu) is asking you to do of course.

Dynamic Qigong is something which seems to be easily dropped by practitioners simply because it is hard to do and can be quite tiring. However, Dynamic Qigong has its place in training, at least as far as most people are concerned and especially those who are practising Martial Artists. Apart from the benefits mentioned above, Dynamic Qigong, sometimes called 'Dong Gong', can improve muscular strength on the inside, helping to improve the action of the diaphragm as well as forcing air to the muscles and other tissue so generally improving the health and strength of the skin, muscles, ligaments and cartilage, etcetera.

Care must be taken not to strain the lungs or burst blood vessels; which should never happen under the guidance of a competent teacher. If you get hot and sweaty, then 'good', that is part of the exercise. As stated above, do not walk away and that includes being tempted to take a shower before finishing your routine. Other advice in this book says that you should start clean, in clean clothes, but it is only natural that you will get a little hot or sweaty during exercise.

Breathing Exercises for a Purpose.

<u>Examples.</u>
These exercises should only be performed when needed and should only be practised by those who have a competent and experienced instructor. Each exercise is used to clear specific areas or Meridians. Although not harmful in themselves, they are quite compatible with other exercises within, but could possibly interfere with Qi that is already well balanced if someone were to experiment with them just out of curiosity. Please take qigong seriously: it is comparable with modern drugs which are administered for specific illnesses, only a fool would take drugs selected for someone else's health problems as the side-effects can cause ill-health, if they are healthy themselves. So why do medical Qigong exercises which you do not need to do? As said earlier on in this book, there has been far too much unguided experimentation in the western world, partially because of books on the subject which do not carry warnings, but also because of humans natural curiosity and the urge to dabble in that which they do not understand and have not studied. This is not to say that an experienced instructor, someone who can tell what effects are being made on his own body, can not try the exercises for himself.

Methods:
1. Gathering Qi at the Dantian. Best done standing. Stand upright, feet not touching but close. Relax.
   a. Breathe deeply, drawing the air and Qi down to the Dantian at the abdomen.
   b. As you approach 'full breath' tilt the torso forwards slightly, to about 45 Degrees by bending from the waist and exhale as you do so.
   c. Inhale again as you return to the upright position.
   Repeat as many times as possible without fatigue.

Note: After some time, the abdomen may feel hot. This is due to the gathering of energies there, do not worry. When this stage occurs, with proper guidance the practitioner should be able to store Qi at the Dantian as well as direct it around the body where needed. This is usually guiding the Qi from the Qihai point up to and around the head, down to the fingertips, back along the outside arms and down to the feet, then back to the Qihai point. Six circulations is sufficient.

2. Clearing the Head. (Any posture).
   a. Inhale slowly and concentrate on moving the 'cool' Qi up through the nostrils, over the forehead, over the crown of the head and down to the back of the skull to the Medulla oblongata – base of the skull.
   b. Exhaling slowly, visualise the Qi back up, over the top of the head and back out through the nostrils again.
   c. repeat this exercise three to five times to help clear the head of "fuzzy" feelings.

3. Clearing the Chest and Abdomen. (Standing Posture).
   a. Exhale deeply three times from the mouth to clear the lungs of stagnant air.
   b. Inhale slowly and visually guide the Qi down through the chest to the abdomen, clearing any blockages or negative energies as it goes.
   c. Exhale and bring the Qi back up the abdomen and chest, then back out through the nostrils.
   d. Do this three to five times.

4. Clearing the Spinal Column. (Any Posture).
   a. Inhaling, guide the breath down the front of the body, down to the Huiyin point, then back to the coccyx – base of spine – and up the spinal column, washing as it goes.
   b. Exhale and guide the Qi/breath over the top of the head, down over the forehead and out through the nostrils.
   c. Once the flow of Qi has been detected, the practitioner can do three to five repetitions the above way, then reverse the flow for the same amount of times the other way – back to front, literally.

These Qigong methods are bordering on the Medical Qigong methods, but in traditional Chinese culture there are many common folk remedies. This is because "self help" is a traditional part of Chinese culture, each person being responsible for themselves to a greater degree: this is almost paradoxically opposite to Western culture where from being born people are brought up to rely on the Orthodox Medical System and National Health Service.

Methods such as the above mentioned, as well as Qigong in general, would be a great benefit in relieving the pressures on medical professionals. It may also lessen the trends for people taking drugs, such as aspirin, at the slightest sign of physical or emotional discomfort. Qigong is a great leveller, especially for those who are stressed in today's manic society with excessive work loads, financial strains and social disorders.

Before it can be of greater use though it has to be accepted as a "normal" thing to do, hence it should not only be introduced to medical centres and hospitals but to primary Schools too. If any student readers or readers who are instructors work within either of these environments, either at floor level or management, then how about doing something really worthwhile and getting the proverbial Qigong ball rolling? Get Qigong introduced as a simple self-help exercise in schools and in medical practice.

Qigong to Overcome Fear or Fatigue.
If you find that you are facing a stressful, fearful or fatiguing situation, then the following exercise may be of benefit to you.

This exercise is not to be performed too often and only if you are in or to face such a situation.

Method:
1. Standing. Suddenly make the whole body taught by tightening all the muscles you can, together and at once. Clench your fists, your feet – dig the toes into the ground, brace the legs with knees slightly bent, clench the teeth and tense the shoulders and back. The chest should be slightly concave.
2. Place the tip of your tongue against the upper palate or roof of the mouth, open your eyes wide as though glaring wildly, pull your chin back so that the neck and

upper spine is rigid. As you are performing 1 and 2, take a sharp inhalation through the nose, making the sound like "Hnnng!", breathing deeply to the abdomen.
3. Exhale explosively through the mouth with the sound of "Ha!" at the same time release all tension and relax the body.

Note: This practice, or similar, is also used in hard style Qigong. Additionally, make sure that the body is relaxed and the breath fully exhaled before being struck by a blow, or in a fall. This minimises risk to the internal organs: the lungs are like balloons to a degree when filled with air, so if struck can expand against the neighbouring organs causing damage and shock; another factor is that when fully exhaled, the body concaves slightly and the muscles are contracted, forming a stronger shield of protection.

Increasing Sexual Potency.
This commonly known method helps those who are lacking in their libido and sexual potency. Traditional Chinese Medicine (TCM) has for years recommended this for anyone who has problems conceiving as it is said to help "revive and stimulate the reproductive organs". Hence there are slight variations for male and female practice.
Male Method:
1. Sit on a chair with straight back and relaxed shoulders, but not slumped. The palms should be resting on the knees.
2. Inhale slowly as you bow forwards slightly, visualise the Qi coming up through the ground, through the soles of the feet (Yongquan) and back through heels and up the legs to the genital region.
3. Exhale slowly through the mouth (jaw relaxed, teeth slightly parted) as you straighten up your body guiding the Qi back down to the feet again, over the toes and out into the earth.

Repeat twenty-five times. Best times are after getting up in the morning and just before getting into bed at night.

Female Method:
4. Sit on a chair with straight back and relaxed shoulders, but not slumped. The palms should be resting on the knees.
5. Inhale slowly as you bow forwards slightly, visualise the Qi coming up through the ground, through the soles of the feet (Yongquan) and back through heels and up the legs to the genital region.
6. Exhale slowly through the mouth (jaw relaxed, teeth slightly parted) as you straighten up your body guiding the Qi back down to the feet again, over the toes and out into the earth.

Repeat twenty-five times. Best times are after getting up in the morning and just before getting into bed at night.
Advanced method:

After approximately three months of regular daily practice the practitioner should refine the technique by drawing the Qi up on the in breath:
- Female (Huiyin) and inwards towards the Uterus
- Male (Huiyin) and inwards to the tip of the Penis.

It is not unusual to get some feeling of Qi or even pleasant feeling tingling sensations. Do not be distracted by these. Only if you get any sensations of dizziness, high temperature or other abnormal conditions should you stop, though these are unlikely. In matters regarding sexual potency, or the lack of it, it is wise to consider that quality of diet, lack of exercise and general health can all play a part, as well as any family inherited health problems, consumption of too much alcohol, drug taking and wearing tight clothing (men especially).

On the flip side, someone of average health taking up Qigong, Kung Fu or even Taijiquan, may experience an awakening of sexual desires. This is perfectly normal, especially in younger people. Older people are also prone to this and age is no barrier to sexual arousal. It should be remembered here that a period of celibacy will enhance the natural processes of the body and help the healing and building of a stronger system. In fact a period of celibacy is good at any time in your life, the Chinese say that for men retaining sperm prolongs life, youthfulness and vigour. There are, I am certain, issues regarding essential mineral intake with this, however these have already been dealt with in the book 'Tai Chi Diet: food for life'.

Arm Swinging Qigong.
This exercise is also called 'Hand Swinging' or Li Shou, sometimes referred to in instruction as 'arms swinging like rope' as the arms are allowed to relax completely as the waist is turned, turning the shoulders like a 'T' bar, to which the rope is attached. This analogy describes aptly the importance of letting all tension go from the arms and shoulders.

This exercise helps build resistance to disease and strengthens the system. It is said to have therapeutic effects in the treatment of bronchitis, stomach problems, high blood pressure, anxiety and depression.

Method:
1. Stand upright, relaxed shoulders and waist, arms hanging loosely by the sides. Keep the tongue down on the floor of the mouth, teeth slightly parted. Relax without being 'floppy'.
2. Swing the torso gently from side to side, as though the waist is a Turntable. As you do this the arms must be allowed to swing like loose rope – this should not be a vigorous movement and the hands should neither swing too far nor too high and should not bang against the body. Keep your eyes on the horizon.

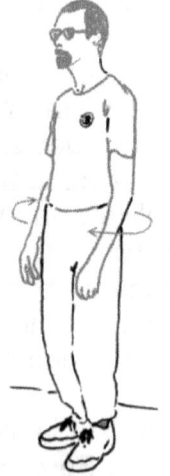

The Start Posture

Knocking on Life's Gates.
Traditional Chinese Pinyin: Tsa Fu Pai.
This is similar to the previous exercise and we often combine these as a pair. In 'Arm Swinging' the tongue is kept down, the Qi therefore tends to build up strength in the two main central Meridians, Du and Ren. When you "knock the two main gates" in this exercise you release any blockages – common at those points – and stimulate the flow of Qi through the central channels, also the tongue is "connected". It is important to keep the waist relaxed and the spine erect, letting the arms swing very loosely with no excess movement, force or over exertion. The hands must make loose or "hollow" fists with either the thumb edge or little finger edge lightly tapping the points on the central Meridians: Dantian on Conception Vessel and Mingmun on Governor Vessel. Be accurate.

Method:
3. Stand upright, relaxed shoulders and waist, arms hanging loosely by the sides. Tongue up on the roof of the mouth, teeth slightly parted.
4. Swing the torso gently from side to side. As you do this the arms must be allowed to swing like loose rope, but this time with loose fists banging lightly alternately against the points Mingmun (lower back) and a couple of inches below the Dantian (outer aspect, of course).

These exercises may be done together, 'Arm Swinging' first and 'Knocking on Life's Gates' secondly, each for the same amount. Repetitions of each exercise can be from eight to sixty-four in all, depending on strength and health. Changing over from the first exercise to the second should be done seamlessly, the instructor having already prepared the class and explaining when 'change' should take place.
Ending the Exercise.

At the end of the exercising, stand quietly with the palms closed and concentrate your mindfulness at the lower Dantian. At this point a little affirmation would not go amiss, perhaps something like, 'I am calm, relaxed and centred', repeated several times. This quiet standing should be done for at least a few moments after every exercise session, the practitioner also reflecting on how well he or she has done, on how much the session has improved their quality of life, health, mental state and general robustness.

Meditations.
The Art of Thinking to not think.

Another subject closely related to qigong is that of meditation. A saying that I recall from my studies of Indian Arts (Yoga, Meditations and Pranayama) is the famous, "An hour of meditation, an inch of Buddha!" This saying tells us that the more time we spend in meditation the more enlightened we will become. This is because the human mind is prone to "chatter", as the psychologists call it, many thoughts, often unrelated, constantly entering our minds and filling our heads with what can only be described as worthless "clutter". The adjective "worthless" is used here because these thoughts are transient, therefore unresolved. Anything which enters one's mind and is unresolved is just wasting time, space and energy, as well as running the risk of causing stress through mental overloading. If a problem exists that is causing the bearer trouble, then contemplation should be employed, concentrating on this order:
1. What is the problem?
2. What are the elements that make it up?
3. Where do these elements come from?
4. Can any of the elements be solved by me?
5. What is the first step that must be taken?
6. When or how can I arrange to take that step?

Contemplation is a form of meditation in respect of focus. Focus eliminates ' mental chatter'. When we get far too much mental chatter this can contribute greatly to stress – the condition of overloading the mind with more problems than it can handle, a mild form of breakdown; just like overloading a car's engine causes a breakdown. Mental Breakdowns are not signs of madness or even inferiority, just in case you are worried. They are normal. Life, especially in "civilised" areas, more especially in City areas, can be very, very stress inducing, especially as one human often transfers their problems on to another by means of involvement, displacement or just plain aggression. Taxes, cost of living, transport and travel, television and other media (they can bring noise, violence, bad news, etcetera to already stressed minds) all contribute. This is why Meditation is so important, especially in built up areas where stress is felt the most. You may notice that people who are lucky enough to live in remote areas or beautiful countryside, hardly ever seem to suffer from stress. This is also why so many hundreds of thousands of Ex-Pat's move to more "laid back" countries like Spain; not just for some sunshine!

Qigong Meditations.
Here are a few useful Taoist Meditations that will help get you started. There are many others to be found if you look around, or search on the Internet using search key words such as 'Taoist meditations', 'Qigong mediations', 'Qigong Cohen', etcetera.

Counting Meditation
1. Begin by lying comfortably on your back.
2. Adjust your mindset to prepare yourself.
3. Exhale fully to clear the lungs of stale air.
4. Count 4 as you breathe in deeply, expanding the abdomen as you inhale.
5. Hold the full breath for a count of 1
6. Exhale for a count of 6.

Repeat this for 8 cycles if unfit, 16 cycles if reasonably healthy. Increase to 16, 24, 32, 40 and so on (adding 8 each week) as you progress. Continue for at least six months to one year. After one year you can increase the breath count to 6-2-8.

Affirmation No. 1.
Think about an affirmation such as, "With this in breath I am getting stronger and wiser" for the inhalation sequence. Then find another for the exhalation sequence, such as "I am expelling ignorance and all weaknesses". These should be

thinkable within the time you breathe in or out. Repeat as many times as possible.

The important thing about affirmations is that you say it and mean it. Be firm and positive. You have the power to change.

Affirmation No. 2.
Seated or standing.
Exhale to clear the lungs of stale gasses.
1. Inhale as you say to yourself, "My body is strong like a mountain."
2. Exhale as you say, "My mind is clear, like a flowing mountain stream."

Affirmation No. 3.
This is a very old affirmation, possibly not Taoist, but used by many psychologists and psychiatrists over the years. Let us go with the Taoist concept of 'If it works, use it. If it does not work, forget it!'

1. As you inhale and exhale slowly, say to yourself, "Every day, in every way, I am getting better and better!"

Affirmation No. 4.
If you have an injury or health weakness, concentrate on the subject or area.
1. For Injury: As you inhale, visualise healing energy coming into your body and to that injury, making it better with every in breath you take.
2. As you exhale visualise that injury leaving your body.
3. For Health Weaknesses: As you inhale say to yourself, "My health issue is getting better and healing"
4. As you exhale visualise that health issue leaving your body.

Affirmation No. 5.
Healing Qi is a very important aspect of Qigong practice. It is by healing that we grow stronger and can help those around us. In this affirmation we learn to build up the power of our Qi and ability to transmit it to others. This should be done as part of a pre-designed programme of training for the Healing Skills, including as a preparation, 'Opening the Energy Channels', as well as other exercises.

Stand or sit with good posture in a dust and fume free darkened room. A dim light should be behind you, or a candle in front of you, but not close and do not look at it directly. Exhale and clear your lungs.
1. As you inhale slowly, visualise Qi entering your Third-eye point - Xuanguan – (Pineal Outlet). Say to yourself mentally imaging, "I am a healer, absorbing healing Qi".
2. Follow the bright healing Qi in as it enters through the Xuanguan point, flows down to the Tanzhong centre, then continues down to the abdominal Dantian.
3. As you exhale, visualise the healing Qi flowing from the abdominal Dantian, up through the armpits, along the arms and out through the palms of the hands – the hand 'wellspring' point, P9 – thus opening your healing powers and ability to transmit healing Qi to others.

It is again important to be positive, seeing yourself achieving your goals. One method which is popular is to see yourself in a dark room, shining with healing Qi, your bright blue Aura is surrounded by white with glowing turquoise and gold outer sparkles. These are the colours of healing, enlightened spirit and purity.

Dantian Meditation.
The sole purpose of this exercise is to build up Qi at the body's most major energy centre, the central distribution point that I liken to the battery on a motor vehicle.

Method:
Stand, sit on a chair, cross-legged with a straight back, or lying down if ill, overweight or convalescing. Place the hands on the

knees or lap, palms up, fingertips touching thumbs, if you are seated. If standing, close the hands lightly. If lying down, follow the Lying Posture guidelines.
1. In your mind's eye, see a stream of white or bright blue-green Qi entering your body as you inhale. Follow this 'stream' to the Dantian.
2. Exhale and keep the 'fresh Qi' at the Dantian.
3. Build up the lower Dantian in this way without breaking concentration.

After a while you may feel heat building up in the abdominal centre. This is natural and a good sign that you are building up the strength of your Qi and the capacity of the lower Dantian.

Speaking of Dantian power: Many years ago, around the 1980's, a man called Terry O'Neill ran a magazine called 'Fighting Arts International'. Terry invited me to send in an article, so I sent one about Qigong. The magazine was full of big macho men in Karate Gi's striking aggressive poses and describing how they mutilate opponents. So, at the Editor's behest, I submitted an article about how I saved my baby's life using Weiqi or Ch'i Expression. Shortly after my second daughter Jane was born, her Qi started to fade and she overslept. It got to point over two or so days when I suspected that if neglected her Qi flow would just stop and she would become another unexplained 'cot death'. The magazine article described how I rested her limp little body across my abdomen so that her Dantian aligned with mine and then gathered my Qi at my Dantian. I then "jump started" her system with a direct Qi transfer. This worked well and she made good recovery over that evening; she is now 26 and living in Finland. Curiously this article did not stir up the ridicule or disbelief that at first expected from these "macho men", most of whom studied traditional Karate. Instead it was apparently well received and Terry (a very gently spoken, genuine and nice man) invited me to send anything else in I liked and it would be published without question! The following articles on Qigong really formed the foundations for this book. Recalling that brings a warm smile to my face. Thanks Terry, hope you are well and prospering! There are enough examples here for most people, so onwards.

Advanced Qigong

This is a specialist subject and really not something I feel can or should be included in a book for general resale. There are aspects, such as Dim Mak (the skill of striking acupoints and causing damage) that in this society of mindless violence and crime is best left solely to responsible Masters. There are other aspects, such as Medical Qigong, which are also obviously best not tampered with by amateurs, no matter how well meaning they may be.

In terms of Qigong and healing we can use an analogy. Would you trust your health and fitness advice to come from a street sweeper, a solicitor, a factory machine operative, office clerk or a general shop assistant? Of course not. You would only go to a specialist, someone who has trained from the basics up. Good, so you definitely would not think of trying to practice advanced Qigong, or any other thing with which you are not familiar and do not have a teacher for, from a book or video!

Another book which I am more than happy to recommend is that by Shih-fu Wong, Kiew Kit, 'Qigong for Health and Vitality'. Shih-fu Wong was the first master I came across that echoed the same well informed knowledge of Qi and Neigong that my Old Taoist Master, Shih-fu Soo did, including Qi expression, healing over distance, etcetera. Shih-fu Wong is also a very highly respected teacher of traditional Shaolin (pre Wushu).

Advanced Qigong stems from basic Qigong practice, just like an apple tree comes from a small seed and grows over many years bearing much fruit; with care, nurturing and knowledgeable pruning. A student of Qigong must first of all understand what it is that he or she is undertaking, including the length of committal. Once the basics have been taught they must be mastered; to 'master' implies that one knows the subject and can practice it without fault or effort; overcome all obstacles, be in command of the subject. Only a fool would want to jump in the deep end of a pool if they could not swim. There are no short cuts, as stated before. The only way to become efficient at Qigong is to start with the basics, master these and then slowly work your way up.

Section 2

TIANDIDAO
天 地 道 拳

八 段 錦
BADUANJIN

The Eight Strands of Silk Brocade

(Pa T'uan Chin)

New (safer) Standardised Sets

TIANDIAO
天地道

八段錦
BADUANJIN

The Eight Subtuts of Silk Brocade

(Pre-Han Chin)

Movement-Standardised Sets

Baduanjin – Eight Strands of Silk Brocade.

Baduanjin, which literally translates as 'eight silk brocade', has always been a very popular exercise in China. Its unusual name derives from the fact that the Chinese character for silken brocade 'jin' also has the archaic meaning of a 'set of exercises composed of different movements'. Hence the title eight pieces of silken brocade can be interpreted more accurately as an exercise composed of eight sets of movements. There is another belief stemming from popular folk lore, one which says the Chinese people would normally have a "best suit of clothes", usually decorated with embroidered designs embroidered from silk. When they put these on it made them feel good, hence this feel good factor also relates to the wonderful effects of Baduanjin.

Below is a potted history of Baduanjin. Thanks and reference must be given here to the many people who have helped create this more accurate history and place their findings on the Internet and especially Wikipaedia, a very useful part of the public domain Internet. This modern communication method has helped me and many others to fill in the gaps in the history and development of this very noteworthy health routine, so limiting misinformation and enabling globally shared education.

History and Development.
Baduanjin has a written history of over 800 years. During this period of time, many modifications and innovations have been added to the original form. Although the variations are numerous, they can be broadly categorised into themes related to the seated and to the standing postures, with the latter further sub-divided into the Northern and the Southern styles. The Set included in this book is that known as 'The New (safer) Standardised Set', this belonging to the Tiandidao (Way of Heaven & Earth) school of practical Taoist Arts.

There has been, and still remains, some uncertainty about the true or exact origins of Baduanjin; many texts and manuscripts have been lost or destroyed over the years and stories passed by spoken word can be altered unwittingly or confused with other folk lore, therefore loosing the original facts or accurate detail. Although Chinese developed health routines date back as far as 770 - 221 BC (Before Christ) and even further, Baduanjin is thought to have been created as a stand-alone set of exercises around the Sung (Anno Domini 960 - 1279) and Ming Dynasties (1368 – 1644). According to modern research and popular belief, the Eight Strands of Silk Brocade, or Baduanjin (八段錦) was said to be developed by General Yue, Fei (Trad. Chinese: 岳飛; simplified Chinese: 岳飞. (Born March 24, 1103 – died January 27, 1142) who was a very famous General in the Sung Dynasty (AD 960 – 1279)

General Yue was a Chinese patriot and Nationalist military leader who fought for the Southern Sung Dynasty against the Jurchen armies. Since his political execution by Chun Kui, General Yue has evolved into the standard model of loyalty in Chinese culture. He also developed Eagle Claw (Yīng Zhǎo 鷹爪) Boxing for use by his enlisted soldiers. The Officers of his army used his other famous and much loved creation, Xingyiquan (Chinese: 形意拳; Pinyin: Xíng Yì Quán; Wade-Giles: Hsing I Ch'üan) is one of the three major 'internal' (Nèijiā) Chinese Martial Arts, also known as 'The Sister Arts' as they are Internal and the three mainstream styles.

The Northern style of Baduanjin, first known publication in China in 1917 by Lian Pu and Jiang Tie Ya, who were both students of the Quing Hua University at the time. Their useful written reference states that an old man from the town of Zheng-Zhou (in Henan) taught these exercises to Lian Pu who in turn passed it on to Jiang. In their version the sequence of movements is:

1. Push the Sky.
2. Draw the Bow.
3. Separate Heaven and Earth.
4. Looking Behind.
5. Search the Clouds and Ground (Tail Wagging).

6. Touching the Feet (Scoop the Stream).
7. Punching with Tiger Eyes.
8. Lifting the Feet (Stand on Tip-Toe & Shaking)

This is one of the earliest references to Baduanjin and since then many variations of the exercises have been created and many variations in order of practice too. As far as this author is aware, there have never been any solid or reliably expert opinions published as to why the order of any given set was laid out that way. It can be guessed that this may be something to do with the creator's knowledge of Qigong and Acupuncture; medical theory of either an individual or a school. However, it is often agreed that the first exercise should be 'Push the Sky', as this has both an awakening effect and a levelling effect on some of the major functions.

Jian and Lian gave their own personal explanation as to the effect of each exercise – I use the names found in the Tiandidao Set to avoid confusion:

1. Two Hands Push the Sky. Regulates the San Jiao (Triple Heater), promotes the dispersing function of the lung, normalises the stomach function and spleen, helps slimming (through digestion and waste elimination), preventing spinal curvature (stoop). Also has effect of improving the function of the spine and preventing and treating cervical spondylartritis periarthritis of shoulder and scoliosis.

2. The Horseback Archer. This exercise can expand the chest, relieve functional disturbances of the lung-Qi, and limber up arms and shoulders; prevent and treat diseases in the neck and shoulder, pain in lower back and leg.

3. Separate Heaven & Earth. Regulates the function of the stomach and spleen, promoting digestion and removing food stagnancy.

4. Looking Behind You. This exercise is said to "remove five kinds of consumptive diseases and seven kinds of general impairment". It is said to "enrich the essence and blood, tranquillize the mind and replenish plentiful essence to the Zang-fu organs so that five kinds of consumptive diseases and seven kinds of impairment are removed".

5. Search the Ground and Clouds. Said in TCM to eliminate the Heart-fire (excess emotion, etc.). This movement has calming effect, mainly used in TCM for neurasthenia and irritability. It is also claimed to improve the motor function of the waist and knees.

6. Bend to Scoop Water from the Stream. Strengthens the Waist, it is used in the treatment of lumbago, promoting a smooth flow of the Qi of the urinary bladder channel and strengthening the defensive energy to protect the integument and musculature against external pathogens so no disease occur (Preventative Medicine).

7. Slantwise Punching with Tiger Eyes. This is said to prevent diseases in the neck, shoulder and lumbar region and for increase physical strength. It improves the power of the chest muscles, shoulders, the biceps and triceps, forearm muscles and fingers, the lower back and legs (especially in the advanced Set). It also induces a strong flow of Qi in all the six main energy channels of the arms, especially the Yin.

8. Stand on Tip-Toe and Shake. Reduces blood pressure, regulates the energy and shakes the internal organs into place. Relaxes and refreshes at the end.

Styles & Comparisons.
There are too many variations of Baduanjin to include in this book although the Tiandidao version is closest to that above, if you just swap numbers 2, 3 and 4 around. Indeed the main

function of the Baduanjin herein is to support those with reference material who are learning the New (safer) Standardised Set of Tiandidao or who already practice a style of Baduanjin but would like to try something different. Included here for reference and interest of the keen student to draw information and historical fact from is a table of comparison of some of the main Sets known world-wide; there are many and I personally came across fourteen common variations during my studies of Baduanjin, and that was in the 1980's, so with availability of world-wide book shopping, Internet and contacts, there are probably many more to be found now.

Key to Table:
Tiandidao = TTT.   OTS = Old Taoist Set.
CLF = Choy Lay Fut.   O.Trad. = Old Traditional.

	TTT	OTS	CLF	O.Trad.	O.Trad.	O.Trad.
1:	Push Sky	Push Sky	Push Sky	Push Sky	Push Sky	Push Sky
2:	Sep.H&E.	Archer	Archer	Archer	Archer	Archer
3:	Look Behind	Scoop Stream	Sep.H&E.	Sep.H&E.	Sep.H&E.	Sep.H&E.
4:	Archer	Look Behind	Look Behind	Look Behind	Look Behind	Look Behind
5:	Search Ground...	Shake.	Search Ground...	Search Ground...	Search Ground...	Side Bend?
6:	Scoop Stream	Search Ground...	Scoop Stream	Scoop Stream	Scoop Stream	Slantwise Punch
7:	Slantwise Punch	Slantwise Punch	Slantwise Punch	Slantwise Punch	Slantwise Punch	Search Ground?
8:	Shake.	Sep.H&E.	Shake.	Shake.	Shake.	Scoop Stream

The items marked with '?' are through uncertainty that they are exactly the same exercises: e.g. In the last Set marked under O.Trad. (Old Traditional), Side Bend could be a variation which looks like a completely different exercise. Likewise, in the same Set, number 7 is originally called 'Bend, Stretch and Scoop', which again is likely to be a different variation to the mainstream Sets. The set which appears to be radically different is The Old Taoist Set (OTS).

Disagreements and differences not only exist in the order of the sections but in what they are thought to do as well. For example, in many of the common sets it is thought that Push the Sky regulates the Sanjiao or Triple Heater, but in one Set they say it affects the Lungs. Below is another Table outlining the two schools of thought on this subject.

Sequence Comparison Table.
Key: Sp. = Spleen.   Liv. = Liver.   Kid. = Kidney.
L. Intest. = Large Intestines.   G.B. = Gall Bladder.
All refer to Energy Channels and their functions.

	Some Common Sets		One Old Taoist Set	Direction
1.	Push Sky	Sanjiao	Lungs	N.W.
2.	Archer	Lungs	Liv. Kid. Skin/Bone, L. Intest.	N.
3.	Sep. H & Earth	Sp/Stom	Back/Spine/Kidneys	W.
4.	Look Behind	Kidneys	Liv.G.B./Eyes/Weight	E.
5.	Search Ground	Heart	Sexual Organs	S.
6.	Scoop Stream	Kidneys	Spl./Pancreas, muscle & digestion	N.E.
7.	Punch/Glare	Liver Qi	Lungs/Nerves/Digestive	S.W.
8.	Shake	Restore	Liv./G.B./Heart/Nerves	S.E.

Whether or not the sequence, or each exercise, does what is claimed of it in terms of Qi flow or enhancement, I do not know for sure. Feedback from other people has stated that they have had better effects from the Tiandidao New (safer) Standardised Set than they have from others; at least one man saying, "I had never felt my Qi before!" This sequence works well, but I shall leave it to the medical Qigong Scientists to explain the whys and wherefores of it. This table is included herein purely for scholarly interest and study and should in no way distract the average practitioner from what is a truly magnificent form of exercise and its main purpose, to improve health.

Research.
In China over the past few decades much research has gone into Traditional Medicine, in particular Traditional Chinese Medicine (TCM). The Chinese have not ignored the many time proven aspects of TCM but have used them as a solid foundation for further research and development. Such aspects as Qigong and Qi Expression, Weiqi or ("Way-chee"), have been combined with surgery to great effect. In one documented hospital operation, a Qigong Master directed his Ch'i to specific acupuncture points on a patient, without physically touching the patient, to numb the area that the surgeons worked on. The operation was successful and the patient felt no pain. This is not fiction, it is fact. This is science in the broader sense and science which is 'hands on', so to speak, not 'remote'; e.g. looking at a segmented subject through a microscope; even if that does have its place sometimes. It is not the kind of medical and impersonal experimentation of the orthodox (western clinical medicine) kind that proves the effectiveness of Qigong, it is the hundreds of years of planned personal and inter-personal trials, expert experimentation, interpersonal information exchange (correlated statistics) and an undisputed profound success that has made Qigong so popular as a healing/health improving exercise. Baduanjin remains one of the leading exercises to be recommended to patients, or recommended as a preventative method; second only to the longer Forms of Taijiquan.

A small but significant percentage of Western medical practitioners, perhaps realising how limited the orthodox system is, especially in the field of treating the whole person, are currently becoming aware of the immense depth of practical and well founded practises within TCM. Many western medical practitioners are thwarted though by the "insurance factors" and the Code of practice under which they train and work; these limit them to what Orthodox Medicine has decreed "safe" for them to practice; truly ironic as many thousands of patients are killed by drugs, surgery or contracted hospital infections every year!

While we are waiting for the western practises to even begin to catch up with both modern and ancient Chinese Medicine, we can make our own informed choices. There is an old Greek saying which I often use, "Physician, heal thyself!" In TCM the most important factor of health is staying healthy and avoiding imbalance, maintaining equilibrium, in other words. This is exactly what TCM has, over the past five thousand years encouraged people to do. Ultimately there is only one person who is responsible for your health, you! This "encouragement" to look after one's self is usually by combined methods of diet, exercise (Qigong and Taijiquan or Gong-fu) and common sense; common sense is practical knowledge combined with perceptive calculation which may ring the proverbial 'warning bells' and which *should* stop humans from doing something potentially harmful.

General Advice.
Will it work? By practising Baduanjin on a regular basis you will be able to judge the results yourself. It will have similar effects for everyone of reasonable health; depending upon their state of health and general conditions in the first place. One thing is for sure, by itself it is both harmless and beneficial, has no nasty side-effects and can only improve your overall health, energy levels and internal fitness. All you have to do is find someone who can teach it correctly, safely and advance you through the various stages.

What essentials must I have?
You must firstly have the will to start. Will power, 'I' ("Yee") in Chinese, is the driving force. Discipline your mind and you can control your body. When practising Qi-gong you must empty the mind of distractions, stop thinking and feeling in the normal sense. We must learn to be empty and relaxed. To begin with you will find this difficult as there is posture and breathing to concentrate on. Your mind's will must be trained to come back into focus on what you are doing until all these things become a subconscious good habit.

Are there any dangers?
There are dangers to anything if tackled recklessly. The areas that could be problematic or most apparent, disregarding personal error, from the incorrect practice of Pa Tuan Chin are;

- Holding in a full breath, especially as you twist or bend. There may be times when the breath is held for a second or so, but always when the body is upright and the internal organs are not cramped.
- Doing bending or twisting exercises if you are pregnant, have ulcers, a swollen appendix, or intestinal problems of such a nature that the exercise might cause stress or bursting, further twisting or strain on stitches from recent operations, etcetera.
- Doing the exercises too quickly and causing a twist, pull or strain of a muscle or tendon or loss of balance and falling over. The exercises should be done slowly and relaxed (not floppy or sloppy) with attention to posture and avoidance of strain, sinking the weight downwards.
- Shih-fu Chan advises that Qigong can exacerbate imbalances, especially in character or mental health, so correct practice and proper instruction are essentials.

Times of Training.
With all Qigong,Taijiquan, Gongfu, Yoga and other exercise, you will realise the most benefit if you train regularly every day. The best times of the day are about one hour after sunrise and one hour before sunset. This is when the air is usually fairly still and dust[8] is settled (except during morning/evening rush hours[9]). Another good time is mid-day and midnight, or just before you go to bed to sleep. Always before meals or at least two hours after eating.

---

[8] Including crop spays if you live near fields and farms, brick or cement dust if you are near a building site, etcetera.

[9] Exercising beside or near busy roads means that you will be inhaling large quantities of Carbon Monoxide fumes from traffic.

Conditions.
Always wear sensible clothing and shoes, or bare feet only if your feet, legs and spine are healthy and you are mindful. Loose cotton clothing is more healthy and sensible than other types of attire.

Never train in dusty, cramped or dirty environments as these are obviously detrimental to your health. Get out in a garden, park, on the beach or common land. You might feel a bit self-conscious at first but fear not, others would dearly love to have the confidence to do likewise! Every time you see a film about China or Chinese communities, you will see people of all ages doing some form of exercise every day out of doors. The old men take their caged birds to the park and hang the cage up while they exercise and socialise. The young and old practice different forms of Martial Art (Ch'uan-shu = Chinese Boxing) from Tiger Style to Taijiquan (T'ai Chi Ch'uan = Supreme Ultimate [Tao] Boxing), a graceful looking form of self-defence which uses the attacker's force against themselves. This makes it popular amongst men and women of all ages up to one-hundred!

If you do have to train indoors then try to plan your room so that you have a utility space. That is a space which can be created by moving chairs, etcetera. The ability to have a window open which will let in some fresh, clean air is also essential. Nylon carpet is not good, nor is any other that would create too much dust, static or otherwise hinder pivoting movements of your feet. Try to avoid hazardous objects like glass-doors in cabinets, heavy objects on shelves, etcetera.

Further Advice.
Once you have set yourself a regular time and space for your exercises then stick to it, try to arrange your day around it and not leave it to chance, or as a disposable option – health is not a disposable option! You will feel much better in yourself for having the discipline to adhere to your planned regime.

Never rush your exercises or break off abruptly. Should you be disturbed at any time during your 'work-out' do not panic, rush or fumble. Remain calm, cool and collected. Finish the exercise that you are doing and centre your thoughts and energy just below the navel, then smile and say to yourself, "I am calm, centred and earthed". This will keep your blood pressure lower and lessen the likelihood of your 'flaring angrily' or becoming flustered at the slightest little setback. Why not give yourself a mental 'pat-on-the-back' by way of applause for staying calm and not flustered.

Every time you complete your exercise set, give yourself a mental pat on the back and contemplate how much good you have just achieved. In today's society it is more and more important to take time to recognise that the health work you have just done is not just beneficial but essential.

Stand Up straight.
One thing which will help you to better health is correct posture. When you stoop or slouch major and minor muscles are being strained. Also the internal organs are cramped by leaning forwards. Try not to ignore these facts or leave it until it is too late.

Be aware of your posture as you sit, walk or stand. You should be upright and well balanced with only a very gentle 'S' shaped curve to the spine but not one which causes aches or strain. Use those shop windows again to check how your posture looks as you are walking. Most of all be aware, for example; What do you see most of when you are walking, feet or faces?

Keeping an upright spine is important in Pa Tuan Chin, as it is in general health, especially when bending or rotating. Always keep your head up straight, as though supported from the sky by an elastic rope attached to the top of the skull. If your Shih-fu (Teacher) is well trained and experienced, he or she might have a veritable arsenal of health and exercise techniques which could help many common health problems, but their knowledge of posture will be more detailed and exacting than most people could imagine. See your Shih-fu for any detailed exercises you may require for posture correction, also 'The complete breath' exercise and others that would be beneficial before you learn Pa Tuan Chin. Just to give you a small idea on how important posture is think about cramp. When you cut off circulating blood and oxygen, as well as potential Qi, then you can clearly feel the effects. Cramp usually affects one limb, but imagine the slower and more long term effect of poor circulation, caused by posture, on the internal organs and whole body.

Effects and Side-effects.
Qigong can help many common problems, from colds to insomnia, digestive disorders, arthritis and rheumatism, nervous tension, heart conditions, high blood pressure, and more. Recent research has concluded that Baduanjin is good for Osteoarthritis of the knees and other medical research outside of the UK has found that Taijiquan – with its associated Qigong effects - is also effective for many forms of arthritis, heart conditions, etcetera.

As mentioned elsewhere in this book, new practitioners may feel some when they start practising. Among these could be itching on one spot, tingling, hot or cold effects, sweating (even in later stages as Qigong really warms you up!), mild changes in either physical or mental state (what I call "wobbles"!), waking up at odd times in the night or even feeling sleepy at odd times during the day; especially if you are in a state of shock or trauma, possibly resulting from injury, operations, horrible circumstances or family loss.

Buddhist Vs. Taoist Qigong.
In Buddhism the emphasis is often placed upon the Mind and it is said that the body is just a vehicle to carry the Spirit, Mind and Qi and has limited life. In Taoism the body is emphasised as it is believed that the life we lead whilst we are alive can be enhanced by making the body better, in health and function. Both Buddhists and Taoists should be vegetarian, therefore reducing toxin and poison intake and making the body and mind clearer. The truth is that the body supports the mind and spirit, so nourishing and cleansing the body will, eventually, help us to achieve spirituality. This is the truth of Yin and Yang (Tao).

EXERCISE CHECK LIST

- ✓ IF YOU THINK YOU MAY HAVE ANY HEALTH PROBLEMS CONSULT YOUR DOCTOR or HEALTH SPECIALIST.

- ✓ ANYONE WITH HEART, BACK OR NECK TROUBLES, ET- CETERA SHOULD SEE A COMPETENT DOCTOR BEFORE COMMENCING ANY FORM OF EXERCISE OR TRAINING.

- ✓ FOLLOW EVERY DETAIL OF THE INSTRUCTIONS CAREFULLY.

- ✓ ALWAYS KEEP YOUR BODY STRAIGHT AND UPRIGHT, WELL BALANCED.

- ✓ DO NOT RUSH THE EXERCISES OR TRY TO DO TOO MANY AT FIRST.

- ✓ ONCE YOU START YOUR EXERCISE ROUTINE KEEP IT REGULAR.

- ✓ DEVELOP CONCENTRATION ON ABDOMINAL AND FULL BREATHING AT ALL TIMES.

- ✓ DO NOT OVERINDULGE IN FOOD, DRINK OR SEX AS THESE CAN ALL AFFECT YOUR CH'I AND CAUSE ILLNESS.

- ✓ WILL YOURSELF TO RELAX THROUGH EVEN THE MOST STRENUOUS OF EXERCISES. LEARN TO CONSERVE POWER AND ENJOY YOUR TRAINING REGIME.

- ✓ IF AT ANY TIME YOU FEEL FATIGUED OR FEEL SEVERE PAIN, STOP. DO NOT TRY TO PUSH YOURSELF PAST THE LIMIT OF YOUR HEALTH OR CURRENT FITNESS LEVEL. INJURY WILL ONLY SET YOU BACK.

- ✓ REMEMBER THAT THIS SET OF EXERCISES IS VARIABLE AND THEREFORE CAN BE MODERATED TO SUIT ALMOST ANY STATE OF PHYSICAL HEALTH OR LIMITATION.

- ✓ THE SET WHICH IS ILLUSTRATED HERE IS THE 'NORMAL' OR STANDARD SET. THIS IS FOR THOSE WHO ARE REASONABLY FIT AND WITHOUT INJURY.

- ✓ BEGINNERS WHO MAY HAVE BACK PROBLEMS, STIFF JOINTS AND MUSCLES THROUGH LACK OF EXERCISE, ETCETERA, WILL NEED TO LEARN THE 'BASIC' FORM WHICH IS MUCH SAFER: THIS CAN BE LEARNED BY ATTENDING THE INSTRUCTOR'S WORKSHOPS - SEE 'PTC COURSES' AT END OF BOOK FOR DETAILS.

- ✓ THIS BOOK IS NOT INTENDED FOR USE AS A TEACHING TOOL BUT AS AN AIDE TO SOMEONE WHO IS LEARNING THE SAME SET FROM A QUALIFIED INSTRUCTOR; ONE WHO HAS TRAINED IN THE NEW SAFER STANDARDISED SET OF PTC WITH T'IEN TI TAO. SEE WWW.TTT-UK.ORG FOR INSTRUCTORS IN UK.

- ✓ SEE 'BACK INJURY' BEFORE STARTING

TIANDIDAO
BADUANJIN SEATED
special needs health care

SPECIAL NEEDS

ADAPTING BADUANJIN

Seated Set

BADUANJIN FOR THOSE WHO CANNOT STAND

The beauty of these simple exercises is that they may easily be adapted for the very elderly who may be too weak or ill to stand for long periods, those who are confined to a hospital bed or a wheelchair. This Tiandidao Set has been examined and structured for safety and good results. The most important thing here is that some exercise is being done to help maintain a healthier body. In this respect Pa Tuan Chin is better than T'ai Chi Ch'uan and far more flexible, permitting adaptation to special needs. Pa Tuan Chin increases health, healing and elimination of toxic waste, etcetera, by increasing the blood circulation and with it the oxygen, so deep breathing is essential. Whilst you are promoting better circulation of the metabolic system you are also doing several other things. One is to stretch the tissues (skin, muscle, ligament, blood vessels and nerves) and therefore keep them more 'elastic' and also allowing any natural body liquids, oxygen and gasses, electrical or other energies to move and circulate freely. Trapped air/gas or stagnant energy may be moved along and eradicated, thus preventing many common ailments which could lead to a build up and something more serious or complicated.

The adaptation of the exercises is simple but, more importantly, flexible. A hospital bed is more spacious than a wheelchair, for example. Therefore one needs to get into the best possible position that circumstances allow. Fresh and clean air is a must, most hospitals are hot and stuffy places! If confined to a hospital ward, ask to be moved to a spot where there is fresh air available, preferably where you can see some trees and flowers - the psychology of viewed-image, perception, is very closely related to health and recovery. Placing a patient in dull and dingy surroundings is not conducive to good recovery. The so-called 'modern' medical profession has known for years the simple fact that a person's state of mind reflects on their health. Many 'old-fashioned' GP's used to recommend that their patients recover whilst holidaying in the Swiss Alps or even by the sea-side. But nowadays many of the men and women of the medical profession appear on the whole to only care about new surgery techniques or new drugs.

It is of the utmost importance to remember that an exercise which is good for one person may be less beneficial to another. This is a dilemma which the aware and caring exercise instructor may be faced with when in front of a class of ten to twenty-five individuals. For example: being very fit I can do exercise number Five ('5') Searching the clouds and ground', with a good posture, deep bend and no ill effects on my spine or back muscles. However, you, or someone else, may have a slight back condition which makes the "full movements" inadvisable. Therefore your instructor needs to have an understanding of movement relating to injury or limitations and be able enough to advise; if s/he is not capable of this advice then the suggestion must be that of "Don't do it!" If in doubt then leave it out.

A person who has been ill and hospitalised is almost certainly going to be more unfit than someone who has at least enjoyed a full range of daily movements whilst working or in leisure. Extra care must therefore be taken with these patients or those who are simply unfit and less active, overweight (consider the load bearing), elderly and frail or those suffering from physically limiting problems.

IMPORTANT NOTE: Breathing.
In any bending or twisting exercise the practising person should always exhale. Full or expanded lungs can place immense pressure on the other internal organs when you are reducing the space internally by bending or twisting the torso.

Practitioners who are new to exercise, particularly Chinese methods, can breathe in as they extend arms in exercises like 'Horseback Archer' or 'Slantwise Punching', as this will increase oxygenation of the body, improving all cells and functions. Later, when they are feeling stronger, the breathing pattern can be reversed; e.g. exhale when extending arms. Also at this stage increased Qi flow may be felt, such as very warm hands, tingling hands, etcetera. Focusing on the movements and exhaling will concentrate the Qi. *This advice applies to both beginner's sets, seated or standing.*

HOW TO DO THE EXERCISES SEATED

Please Note: The techniques in this section are similar to the standing set but done more gently, or "fine tuned" for the special needs patient. One thing which should remain the same, even if exercises are "cut down", is the will to do better or make bigger movements.

THE SEATED FORM

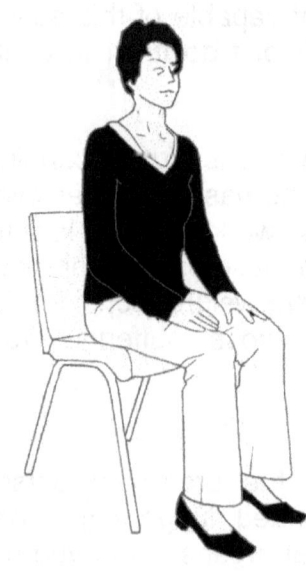

Preparation Posture

Preparation: Sit upright on your chair or in bed with the feet approximately shoulder's width apart. Keep the head upright and spine straight but relaxed (not cramping the diaphragm or lungs), focus your eyes on an imaginary horizon, eight miles away – this helps to keep the head level and upper spine straight. Keep your shoulders and arms relaxed with your hands resting beside you. The expression, 'chest concave', sometimes stated by other Chinese Arts practitioners as a 'hollow chest', simply means letting the tips of the shoulders relax and drop forwards slightly making a slight hollow beside the armpit area.

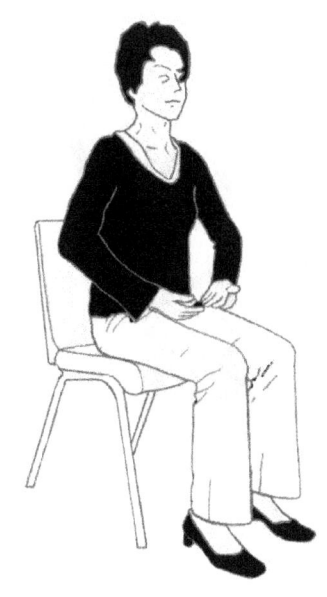 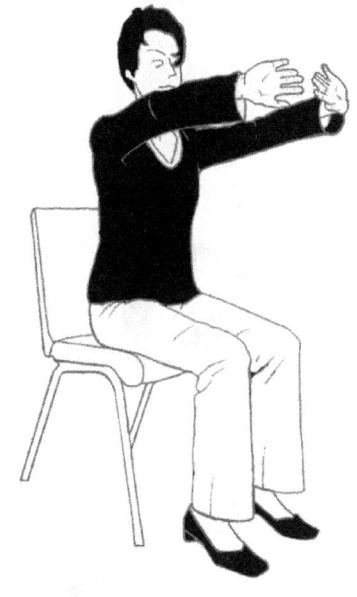

1a.   1b.

1: 'Two Hands Push The Sky'.

Slowly raise both hands, palms up and turning the fingertips inwards (As in Figure 1a). Turn the little-finger-edge of the hands downwards-and-forwards, 'scoop' them forward, outwards and up to above eye level as you take a deep breath, stretch both arms gently but positively forwards to the maximum or as far as personal comfort will allow, stretching the shoulder blades apart (Figure 1b). Slowly bring them back down the same way exhaling at the same time, turning the hands over to rest them by the sides.

Repeat 4 to 8 times in all, smoothly.

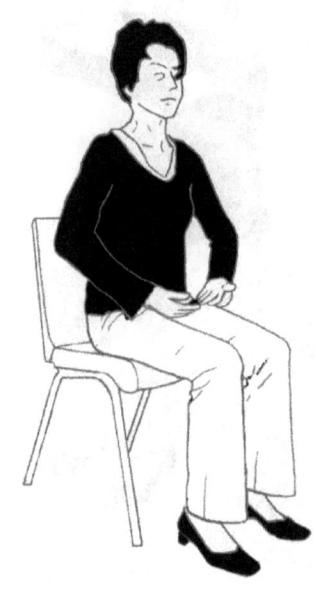 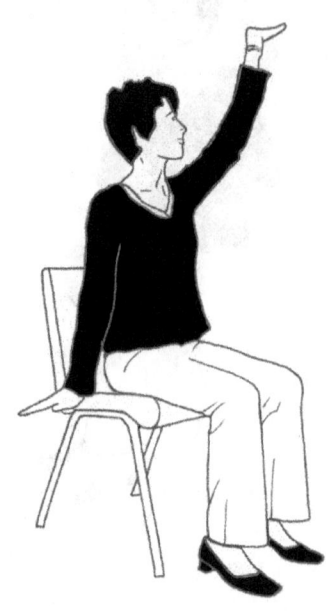

2a. 2b.

2: 'Separate Heaven and Earth'.

Sit upright with your hands by the sides. Slowly raise both hands as before (Figure '2a.') to mid-abdominal height.

Continue smoothly to raise the left hand slowly as high as possible above your head. Simultaneously lower the right hand to behind the right thigh/or push down gently on the bed beside the buttocks/or push down beside the chair. Stretch the two apart, as though pushing apart the sky and the earth. Look at the upper hand if possible (Figure 2b.).

Next, bring them slowly down to the starting position as you exhale and change over as they meet, raising the right hand and lowering the left hand alternately.

Do this 4 to 8 times each side. Relax to finish, hands by the sides (As in the first illustration, 'Preparation Posture'.)

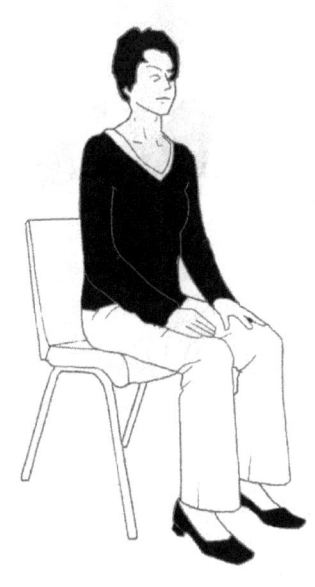

3a.

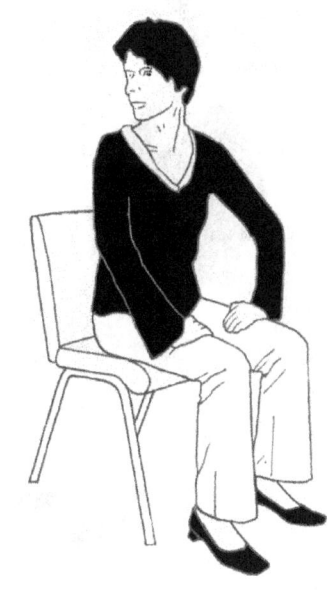

3b.

3: 'Looking Behind You'.

Start as in Figure '3a' with your hands on your legs. Turn both hands inwards, so that your fingertips are facing inward towards each other, your palms resting on the thighs for support. Inhale quietly and deeply without strain.

Slowly turn to peer over the left shoulder (Figure 3b.), exhaling as you turn to look behind you keeping your head and spine upright.

Slowly return to the starting posture as you inhale and look straight ahead, at the imagined horizon. Keep your weight sinking down and the shoulders free of tension.

Repeat this movement to the right.

Repeat very slowly and gently 4 to 8 times each side.

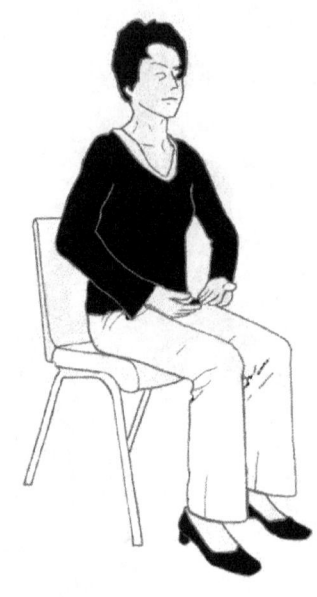

4a.

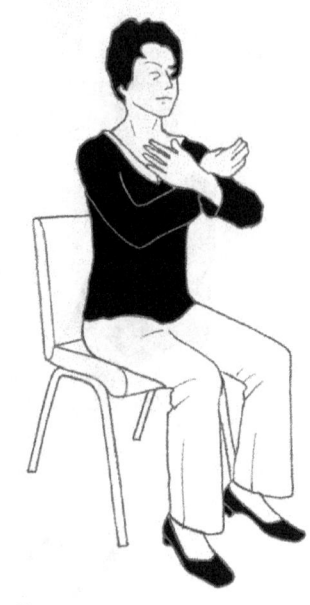

4b.

4: 'Riding on Horseback and Drawing the Bow'.

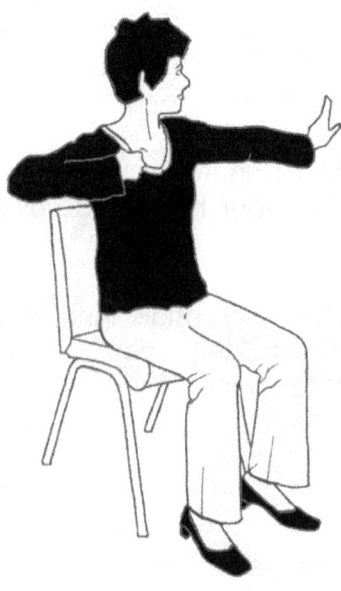

4c.

Prepare as in figure 4a. by turning the palms up, fingertips touching, in front of the abdomen. Bring the hands up to cross in front of the chest - left in front of the right. Look ahead and keep your head aloft (Figure '4b.').

Slowly stretch out the left hand with forefinger and middle finger raised toward ceiling, thumb out naturally and other two fingers curled into palm. Pull the right hand back at shoulder level, fingers curled, as though drawing a bowstring. Look at the left index-finger's nail (Figure '4c.'). As you reach maximum stretch, relax and return to the crossed hands position (As in Figure 5)', but this time with the right hand in front.

Repeat the 'bow pulling' to the right, exchanging left for right in the instructions. Keep the spine straight.

Repeat very slowly and gently 4 to 8 times each side.

Detail:
In Figure 4d, opposite, you can see the detail of the 'Bow hand' position as well as the "flatness" of the line across the shoulders and chest. The fingertips should be pointing up directly to the ceiling, although if this is too much of a stretch at first it can be achieved gradually. This position should provide a really good stretch across the upper chest and throughout the arms without strain.

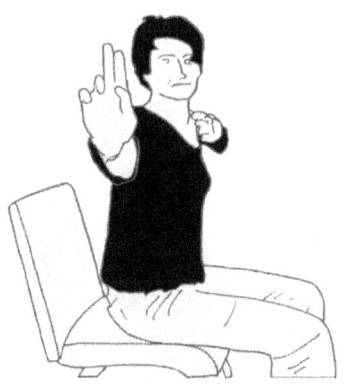

4d. Close-up of Archer Position

5: 'Searching The Clouds and Ground'.

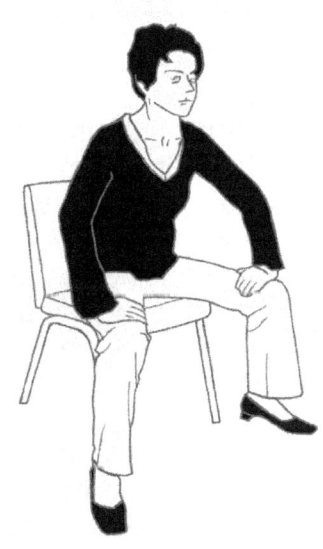

5a.

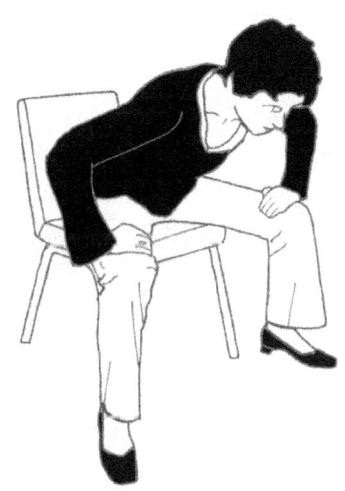

5b.

Preparation is the same as number 1, but then move the feet further apart to enable forward leaning.

Inhale. Place the hands on the thighs, thumbs and forefingers towards the upper thigh (Figure 5a.). Then exhale slowly as you carefully lean forward, just a little at first, looking at the ground/bed (Figure 5b.)

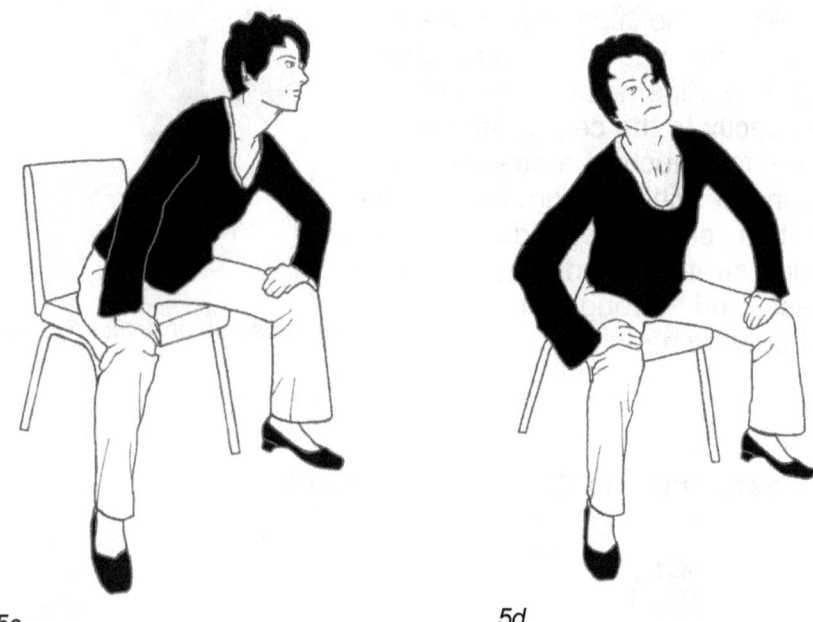

5c. 5d.

Rotate the trunk to the left (Figure '5c.'). Do not lean back directly or bend the neck, you should be at a very slight angle and looking diagonally forward towards the ceiling. Inhale again as you lean back (As in Figure 5c.). The spine is pivoting on the axis of the Lumbar Region, so that the head and upper spine goes to the left and the tail-bone (Coccyx) inclines towards the right, like a wagging tail!

Rotate back the way you came, through 'centre', and look again at the floor as you exhale. Carry on around to the right (Figure 5d.) and repeat the exercise 4 to 8 times in each direction. This exercise is like a gentle swaying from side-to-side in a circular motion.

NOTE: Be extra careful of the neck in exercise 3 & 5 as people who are bed ridden may be in a weaker state physically than those who move around normally. Their situation should be taken as "potentially dangerous" and all movements, exercise or not, thought about carefully. Gentle exercises should be undertaken with a view to increasing strength and mobility carefully.

6: 'Bend to Scoop Water From The Stream'.

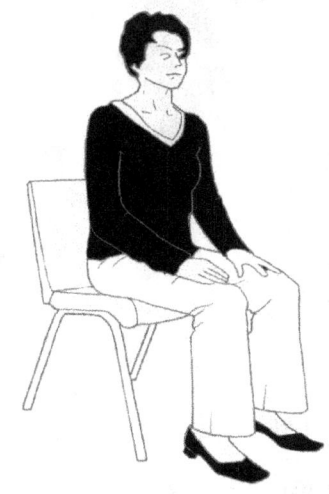

6a. Prepare.

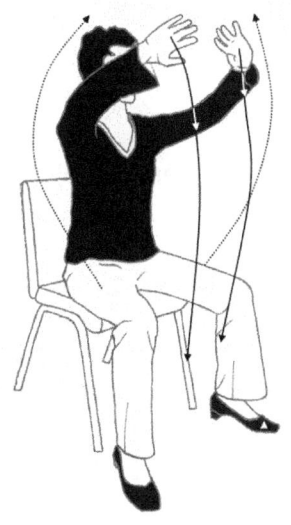

6b. Gather Qi

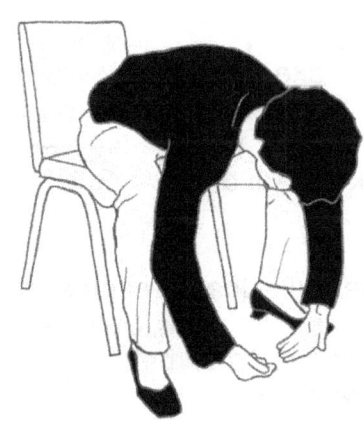

6c. Scoop the Stream.

Preparation is the same position as you should be in when finishing the previous exercise (Figure 6a.) Turn your hands palms up, raise them forwards and upwards (gather Qi) and at the apex – head height – turn the palms over to face downwards again (Figure 6b.) Slowly exhale and pull in the tummy as you bend forwards, (Figure 6c.) keeping the spine stretched forwards and straight. As you reach your lowest point, extend the hands downwards/forwards, as though scooping water from a stream by your feet (Figure 6c again). Inhale as you sit up straight and return the hands to mid-body height, turning the palms upwards; this can be adjusted to suit individual needs.

Note: If the back is weak, the practitioner has backache or other problems which deter them from bending so deeply, then a less deep bend may be done; such as the illustration below (Figure 6d.) Care must be taken at all times so as not to exacerbate any problems but instead gently improve the health and flexibility of the practitioner.

Repeat very slowly and gently 4 to 8 times.

Conditions such as weak back muscles may exist if the practitioner has not done any form of stretching, manual work or bending for a long time, being bed ridden for an extended period will also weaken the back as muscle tone and strength deteriorate when not used; this usually takes months rather than weeks, however, not exercising for just a week or two can have a dramatic effect on muscles and ligaments.

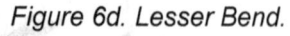

Figure 6d. Lesser Bend.

Any member of the public seeking to take up regimes like this should mentally prepare first of all, followed by gentle warm-ups, then moving on after a week or two to a gentle set of stretches and finally something like Baduanjin – Basic or Seated.

Instructors should fully ascertain the individual strengths and weaknesses of new members coming in to their classes as well as providing such written information and verbal advice as is necessary; including appropriate warnings.

7: 'Punching Slant-wise and Glaring'.

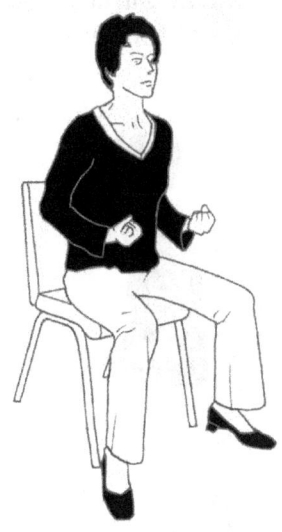

Figure 7a. Forming Loose Fists.

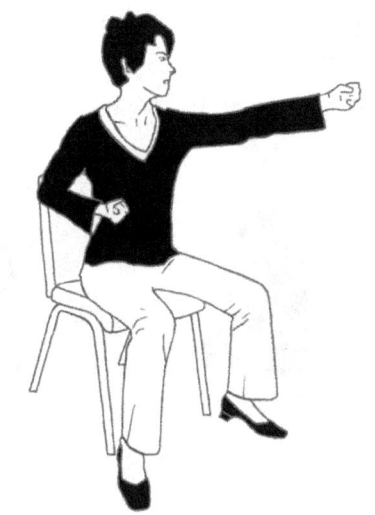

Figure 7b. Punch Diagonally Leftwards.

Prepare for this the same as exercise number one. Bring your hands slowly off your legs and make very loose fists as you turn both hands palm-up (Figure 7a.) in front of the waist – not too close and do not pull the elbows back as this will tense the shoulders! Settle and keep sinking your weight down.

Slowly, punch the left fist outward at a 45 degree outward-and-upwards angle as you slowly punch the fist out to a full stretch (figure 7b.). Keep your head stretched up and the lower spine sunk down and straight. Open your eyes wide, "glaring" at the outstretched fist. Slowly relax the arm as you also exhale and return to the starting posture.

Next, bring the right fist out in the same manner, glaring at the 'eye of the fist' as you extend it fully (Figure 7c.).

Repeat this exercise 4 to 8 times with each arm.

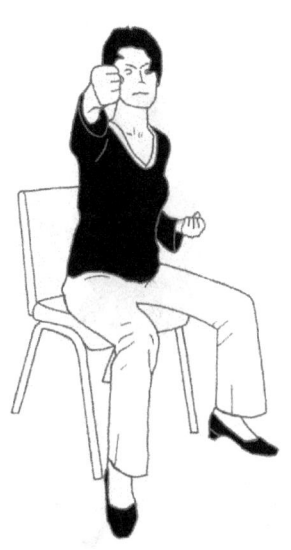

Figure 7c.

8: 'Sit Up Tall and Shake'.

Prepare as in the first exercise. Keep relaxed at all times as this exercise seeks to eliminate tension, so do not tense as you stretch.

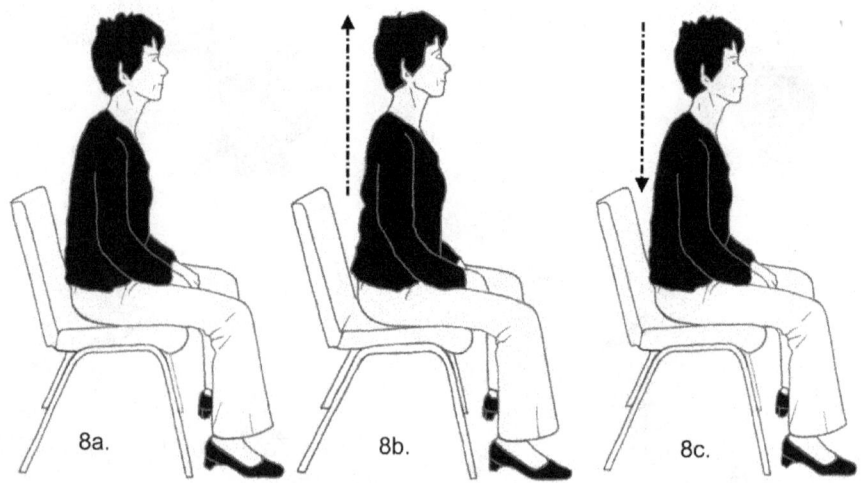

Sit upright and keep the spine stretched straight (Figure 8a.). Inhale and raise the very top of your skull until you feel as though lifted to full stretch by a thread attached to the top of the head (Figure 8b.). Your bottom should be almost rising from the chair/bed, but with no assistance from the feet, hands or legs.

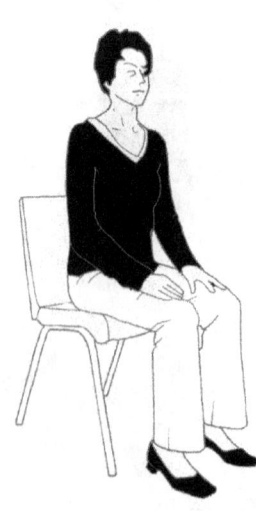

Let the breath escape naturally as you suddenly 'release', dropping the bottom back down onto the chair/bed (Figure 8c.) but keeping the spine straight and without "jolting", just a very *gentle* "bump"; this should have a gentle but positive stimulation of the nervous system.

Repeat 4 to 8 times.

Return after this to the neutral starting posture. Sit quietly for a few moments and contemplate your Dantian.

Conclusion

This concludes the simple but highly beneficial 'Eight Strands of Silk Brocade' for those who are not able to stand. The set can be done two or more times per day, as much as energy allows. As the practitioner feels better, he/she can then increase each of the eight exercises to eight repetitions each, or eight left and eight right (for numbers 2,3,4,5 and 7). Again, the exercise set should be done in full and evenly - that is to say, do not just concentrate on one or two of the exercises alone. They are designed to be most beneficial as a complete set.

There is no age limit and no size criteria. As long as a person is able to move any limbs then there is no excuse for not exercising in such a gentle and health increasing manner. In this light a positive attitude is a must. By a 'positive attitude' it is meant that someone should be in the right state of mind before undertaking exercise. If a person is ill then they should have a strong desire to get better. If a person is unfit, then they should harbour a strong desire to get fit and stay fit. Once the decision has been made to do the exercise then that goal should be extended to include 'regular' in the equation.

The biggest obstacle to overcome from both a teacher's viewpoint and that of the individual is this National Health Service 'care' syndrome. As mentioned earlier in this book, many millions of people are born into this world and brought up to rely on an already overstretched health service. We are all responsible for our own body and even if we rely on the kind help of others to execute daily essentials for us, then we are still ultimately responsible - as long as we are able - to do what we can. If competent teachers of the 'safer' Set can train both the public and members of the health care profession then this alone will cut the future queues at Hospitals and local surgeries; as well as planting more seeds of preventative health care amongst the families of those involved.

TIANDIDAO
BEGINNER'S BASIC STANDING SET
of
BADUANJIN

Baduanjin Beginner's Basic New Standardised Standing Set

The Preparation Posture.
In all standing versions the starting posture is the same. In Chinese Arts which derive from or intermingle with Martial Arts, these are often known by names of animals or association.
The Preparation stance for Baduanjin in the standing form is called 'Eagle Stance' (Figure 'A').

Method:
Stand with your feet together, head raised but not straining the neck. Jaw, shoulders, waist and arms relaxed. Bend the knees very slightly ('keeping the knees soft') and tilt the pelvis slightly down and forwards so that the lower back is straightened. Your eyes should gaze straight ahead, towards the horizon; if you can not see the horizon, imagine it eight miles away as a vague image of a gently curving line.

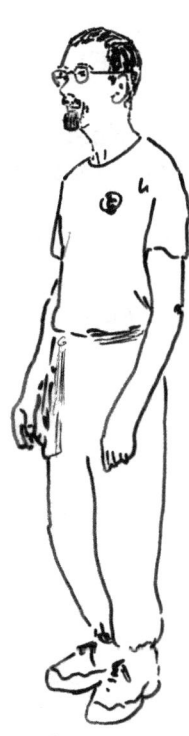

Eagle Stance

Allow yourself time to relax and for the breathing to settle down to a slow, regular pattern. This is the time to do a complete head-to-toe body check:
- ✓ Head upright?
- ✓ Shoulders and arms relaxed?
- ✓ Waist relaxed?
- ✓ Back straight?
- ✓ Pelvis tucked in slightly?
- ✓ Knees slightly bent (unlocked)?
- ✓ Heels close together and toes out?
- ✓ Fingers and hands relaxed?

Once you are happy with your posture then you are set to begin.

THE SIMPLIFIED FORM

1: Two Hands Push the Sky.

This is like stretching when we awake. To begin with this posture removes fatigue and takes in fresh air to stimulate us. It also induces a stronger blood flow in the thoracic and abdominal cavities, thus helping to regulate all the internal organs. There may also be useful side-effects with the muscles and bones of the lower back, waist, upper back, chest and shoulders, helping to correct 'stoop' and improve movements, toning the nervous system at the same time!

THE FORM
Preparation: Stand with the feet approximately shoulder's width apart. Keep the spine straight but relaxed, eyes on horizon. Slightly bend the knees. Keep shoulders and arms relaxed.

1: 'Two Hands Push The Sky'. Slowly raise both hands and turn the fingertips inwards (Figure '1' far left). Turn the little-finger-edge of the hands downwards and scoop them out-and-

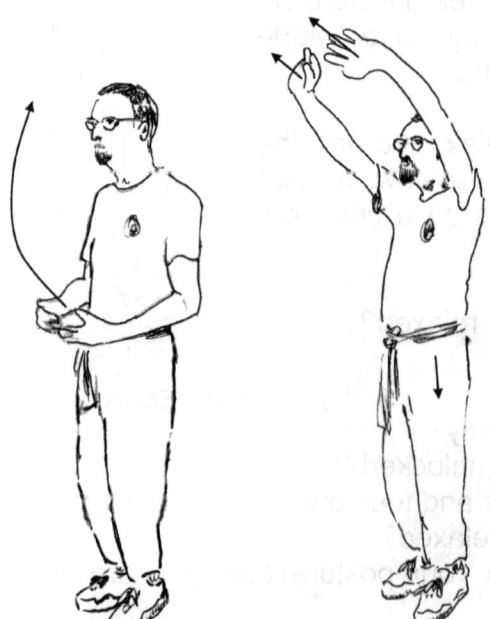

up to above eye level, stretch both arms forwards to the maximum (Figure '2' right). Slowly bring them back down the same way, in a large semi-circle, turning the hands over to rest them by the sides.

Repeat 4 times in all, smoothly and centre the Qi at the Dantian.

2: 'Separate Heaven and Earth'.

This is the second posture or exercise in the Set. This has pronounced effect on the Spleen, Gall and Stomach. It can aid the digestive functions as well as stretching major and minor side-muscle groups. Therefore regularity will help eliminate risk of gastrointestinal disease or aid in the cure of it.

THE FORM
'Separate Heaven and Earth'. Start as in Figure 'A'. Slowly raise both hands, as before (Figure '3', below left). Continue to raise the left hand slowly as high as possible. Simultaneously lower the right hand to behind the right thigh (fingertips outwards on both hands). Stretch the two apart, as though pushing apart the sky and the earth. Look at the upper hand (Figure '4'). Next, bring them slowly down to the starting position - Figure '1' - and change over, raising the right hand and lowering the left hand.

Do this 4 times each side. Relax and centre the Qi at the Dantian to finish, hands by the sides (as in the first illustration, Figure A)

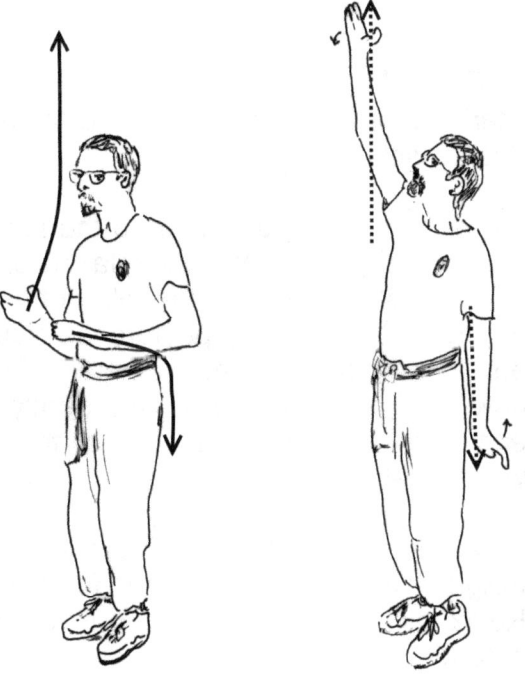

Notes: It is important to keep sinking your weight down as you stretch the hands upwards and downwards. By "sinking" it meant that you tuck your pelvis forward and downwards slightly, as though going to sit; thus straightening the lower spinal column.

3: 'Looking Behind You'.

This obviously has a more pronounced effect on the neck and head region but the small 'core' muscles which aid spine support and turning are exercised here also. When turning the head you are stimulating the muscles of the neck (cervical and vertebra), throat and eyes. Stimulus of the cervical muscles helps to promote health of the brain and systemic nerves. It is also useful to improve equilibrium in patients with Hypertension and Arteriosclerosis. A noted lessening of mental fatigue may be partly due to a refreshing stimulation of the central nervous system. Considering that the general distribution passage of the nervous system runs along the path of the vertebrae, then it is no surprise that this exercise can have a positive effect on the rest of the body and internal functions. For those who have weak Pelvic Floor muscles, exhaling as you turn and consciously pulling in the lower abdominal muscles will help to strengthen these; although this is not strictly speaking Qigong, it does serve to improve health physically and it should be remembered that the physical, physiological and Qi functions of the body work together as one.

THE FORM
Start as in Figure 'A'. Inhale quietly and deeply without strain.

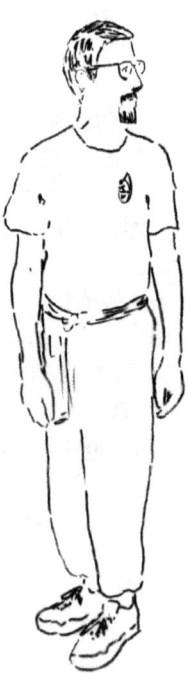

Slowly turn the upper torso to the left, exhale slowly and peer over your relaxed shoulders at the right heel (Figure '5', right). Slowly return to the starting posture as you inhale and look straight ahead. Keep weight sinking down. Repeat very slowly and gently 4 times each side and centre the Qi at the Dantian when finished.

Notes: Keep the spine straight and sink the weight. Do not lean. Do not force the turn. Relax and try to make your movements natural.

4: 'Riding on Horseback and Drawing the Bow'.

The Chinese health practitioners consider the upper-chest (Thorax) region to be second only in importance to the head. This exercise stretches and expands the chest, enhances the activities of the Lungs and Heart, stretches and tones the muscles in the arms, shoulders and armpits. It is known to assist also in the ridding of pathogenic symptoms resulting from negativity or neglect.

THE FORM
Begin by shifting your weight to your right leg. Step out left with the left foot into the "Riding a Horse" stance. Sink the weight down as low as possible.

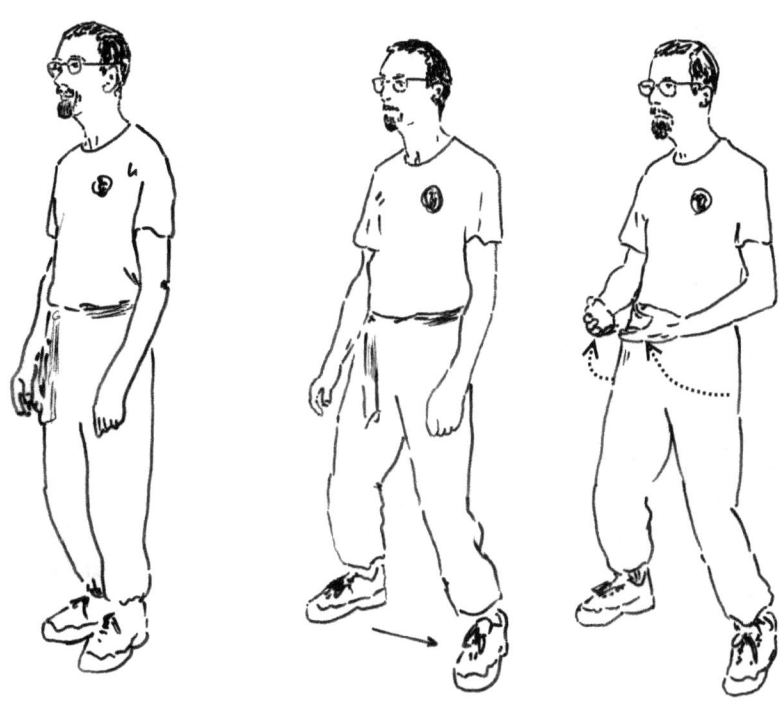

Bring the hands up to cross in front of the chest - left in front. Look ahead and keep your head aloft (Figure '6', centre). Slowly stretch out the left hand with forefinger and middle finger raised toward ceiling, thumb out naturally and other fingers curled into palm. Pull the right hand back at shoulder level, fingers curled, as though drawing a bowstring. Look at the left index-finger's nail (Figure '7', right). As you reach maximum stretch, relax and return to the position as (far left figure), but this time with the right hand in front. Repeat the 'bow pulling' to the right, exchanging details.

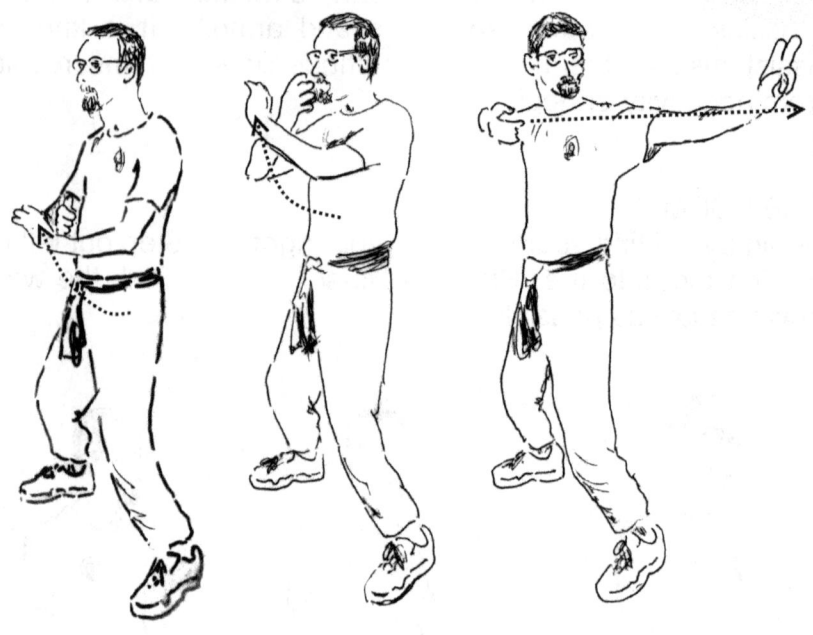

Repeat 4 times on each side. Slide left foot in to end and centre the Qi at the Dantian.

Notes: Keep the spine straight and sink the weight. The head needs to be kept upright so that the spine is as straight as possible. In this, the Standard Set, it is important to remember that this set is for beginners, so maximum postural benefits should be achieved without strain.

5: 'Searching The Clouds and Ground'.

This rotates the spine from top-to-tail with the lower 'lumbar' region being the pivotal point. The Chinese say that this exercise 'removes Heart Heat'. 'Heart Heat' has no accurate description in Western terms, but it is associated with the symptoms of stress and anxiety in Acupressure method. One point where the intrinsic energy (Ch'i) can 'block-up' is on the Governor Meridian at the base of the spine. It also translates as being to do with the sympathetic nervous system. A healthy person may be rid of tensions and stress after a rest. Some people do not shed negativity and daily strains quite so easily. In this case there may be a build-up of tension leading to pathoses - disease forming situation. So this exercise rotates the spine, massages the nerves, releases tension and helps the internal functions.

THE FORM (beware of the spine!)
Begin by shifting your body weight to your right leg and inhale. Step out left with the left foot into the "Riding a Horse" stance. Sink the weight down as low as possible by bending at the knees. Place the hands on the knees, thumbs and forefingers upwards (Figure 8, far left). Then slowly exhale and lean forward, looking at the ground Figure 9, centre). Rotate the

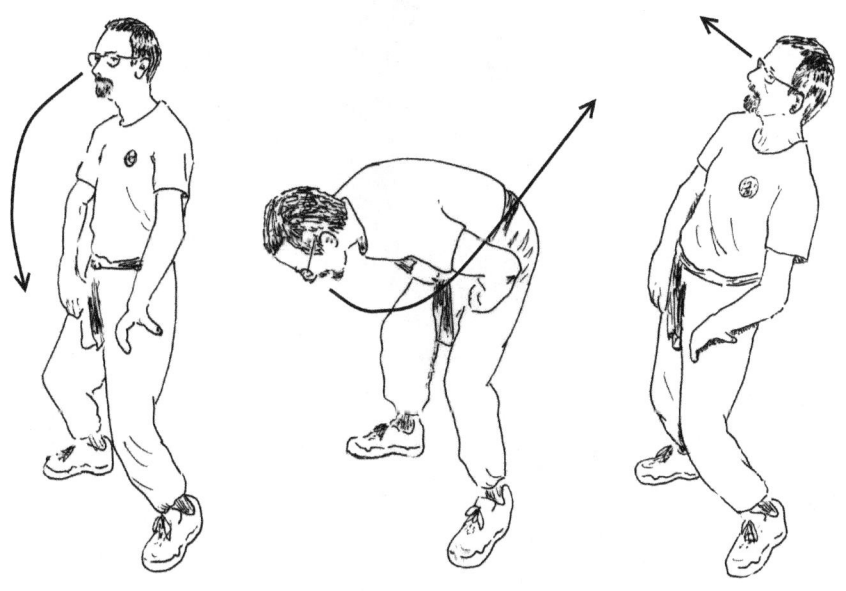

trunk to the left (Figure '10', far right - above). Stop before you are leaning back directly, you should be at a slight angle and looking at the sky or ceiling in front of you at a 45 Degree angle; inhale as you do this. Rotate back the way you came and look again at the floor as you exhale. Carry on around to the right and repeat the exercise 4 times in each direction.

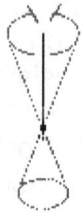

The spine is pivoting on the axis of the Lumbar Region (see inset picture below) in a dual cone shape. The pivotal point is the dot at the 'neck' of the cone, this represents the pivotal point of the spine which is just above the Sacrum – five joined or "welded" vertebra just above the Coccyx – illustration below.

Notes: Never put pressure on the spine by bending it too far backwards or sideways as this can cause rupture of the Discs between the Vertebra!

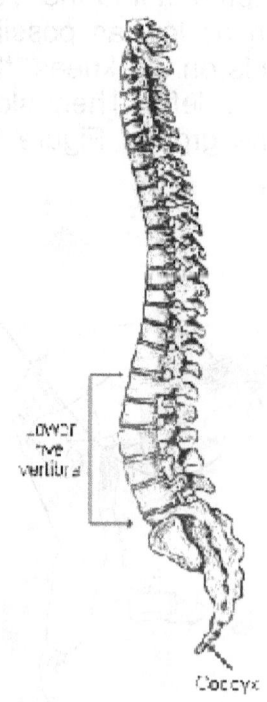

6: 'Bend to Scoop Water From The Stream'.

This exercise has two parts. In the first sequence we bend from the waist and 'scoop' with our hands. Then, in the next part (optional) we raise the arms and "wash" with the Qi we have "gathered". The actions of this exercise strengthen the waist, lumbar, and circulation.

THE FORM (beware of the spine!)
Start as in Figure 'A'. Raise the arms as in Gathering Qi exercise, turn the palms over and start lowering the arms and hands, as though pressing a post down into the ground (Figure '11' left). Slowly exhale as you bend the knees and bend forwards, keeping the spine stretched forwards and straight. As you reach your lowest point, extend the hands downwards, as though scooping water from a stream by your feet (Figure '12', right). Inhale as you stand up and return the hands to mid-body height, turning the palms upwards. Repeat 4 times. Centre Qi at Dantian when finished.

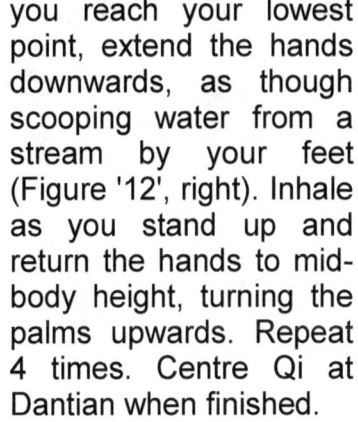

The 'optional' Qi Washing is shown here and is a useful addition to the basic Standard Set. As you return to the upright position, using the legs (not the back!), imagine "washing" with the Qi that you have just gathered, letting it wash from the top of the head downwards, washing away all things negative as it descends through the body and out through the soles of the feet.

7: 'Punching Slant-wise and Glaring With Tiger Eyes.

This exercise increases strength and stimulates the Cerebral Cortex and qi flow through spine and arms.

THE FORM
Begin by shifting your entire weight to your right leg. Step out left with the left foot into the "Riding a Horse" stance. Pull both fists up to your waist as you settle and sink your weight down as low as possible. Keep the shoulders relaxed, chest concave, back and head upright and your eyes gazing straight ahead (Figure '13', below and left). Keep the shoulders and arms relaxed as you let the hands "float" up to waist level and make loose fists (Figure '14', second and third left).

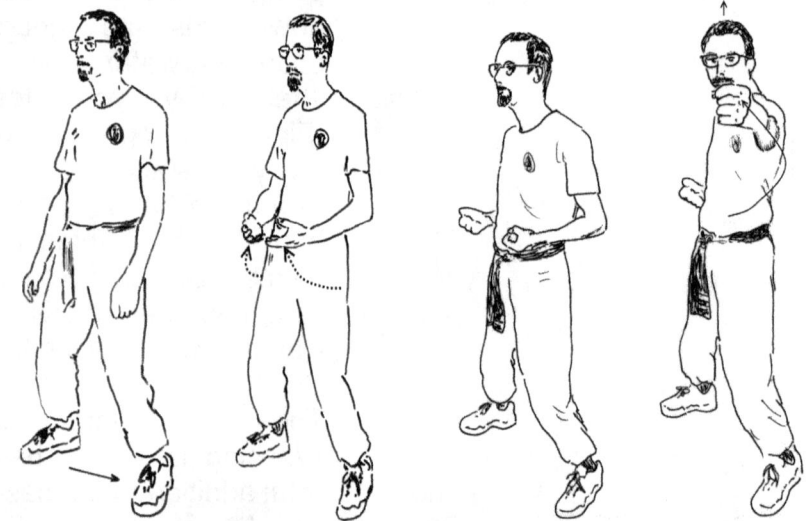

Slowly, punch the left fist outward at a 45 degree outward-and-upwards angle. Keep the head stretched up and the lower spine sunk down and straight. Glare your eyes at the outstretched fist (Figure '15', far right). Slowly relax the arm as you return to the starting posture (Figure '14, second left image').

Repeat this exercise 4 times with each arm. Pull in the left foot to finish. Centre the Qi.

8: 'Stand on Tip-Toe and Shake'.

This *gently* shakes the internal organs back into place and relaxes. It is an ideal way of finishing (closing) and should be followed by a short period of standing still and quietly whilst concentrating on the Dantian (Tan T'ien/Tanden/Hara) point just below the navel.

THE FORM
Starting posture for this is as in Figure 'A'. Stand up on tip-toes (and ball-of-foot) until you feel as though lifted to full stretch by a thread attached to the top of the head. Inhale as you do this (Figure '12'). Let the breath escape naturally as you suddenly 'release', dropping the heels to within one centimetre of the floor *. Repeat 8 times.

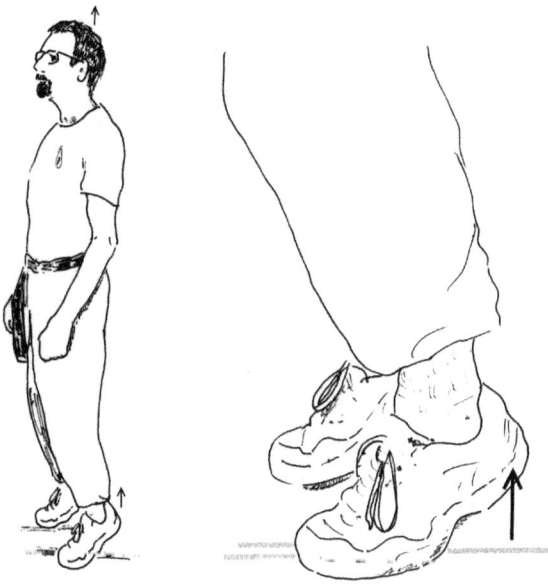

Notes: Do not let the heels 'bump' on the floor as this causes jolting of the spine which is not healthy. The idea is to gently shake the internal organs into place and 'vibrate' them and the nervous systems in a gentle and caring manner.

The Eight Strands of Brocade should be done every day to achieve best results. Its movements at first have to be learned, therefore they will be separate and jerky. When you have learned them you should concentrate on doing all eight exercises smoothly and joined up, like T'ai Chi Ch'uan. You should not be tense when stretching or moving, rather be like a cat when it stretches, lithe and relaxed.

After initially doing the exercises 4 times each on each side, aim to do more. Increase it to 8 times each on each side and do the whole set. When your stamina allows, you can do the whole set more than once. Always do the whole set and do not just take out one or two of your favourites as this may cause imbalanced exercise and will not do you so much good as originally intended.

More Important Advice on breathing:
Inhale and exhale naturally. But when you twist to the rear or sides, or bend sideways or forwards, then exhale.

Never hold your breath while exercising. This is important advice and must not be ignored. Some advice may be repeated in this book, and for good reason; to make sure that it is seen and hopefully followed.

**NEVER DO CH'I KUNG IF YOU HAVE A HIGH FEVER
IF YOU ARE MENSTRUATING OR PREGNANT
IF YOU ARE FEELING DIZZY OR FEINT**

This concludes the basic "Standardised Eight Strands of Silk Brocade" exercise set. This is only the basic form which should serve everyone well. This Form is suitable for young and old, Martial Artists, Gymnasts and all sports-people alike. With regular practice you will notice some quite dramatic improvements to your daily health, an uplift in energy and spirit and the ability to ward-off common ailments.

There are more advanced variations with specific breathing techniques and posture variations for both health and Martial Arts purposes. This set will be of more than enough benefit to most people.

> AVOID THE EXERCISES IF YOU HAVE ANY DOUBT WHATSOEVER AND CONSULT YOUR PHYSICIAN OR KNOWLEDGEABLE (about Qigong and exercises) SPECIALIST!

TIANDIDAO
The New Standardised
ADVANCED BADUANJIN SET

WARNING:
Only for people who are in good physical health, who have no spinal injuries or problems, and have practised the basic Standardised Set for at least one year under qualified instruction.

ADVANCED SET – LEVEL 3.

(1) 'Two Hands Push The Sky'.

This is like stretching when we awake. To begin with this posture removes fatigue and takes in fresh air to stimulate us. It also induces a stronger blood flow in the thoracic and abdominal cavities, thus helping to regulate all the internal organs. There may also be useful side-effects with the muscles and bones of the lower back, waist, upper back, chest and shoulders, helping to correct 'stoop' and improve movements, toning the nervous system at the same time!

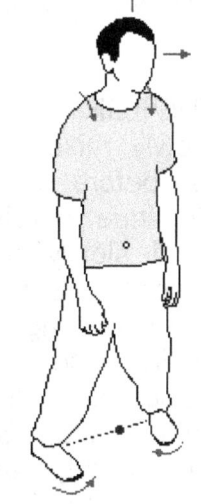

THE FORM

Preparation: Stand relaxed with your feet approximately shoulder's width apart. Keep the spine straight, eyes on horizon. Slightly bend the knees. Keep the shoulders and arms relaxed and natural.

Preparation

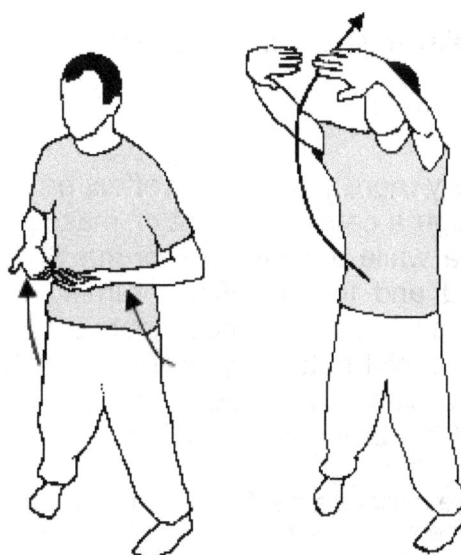

1: 'Two Hands Push The Sky'. Slowly raise both hands and turning the fingertips inwards (Figure '1'). Turn the little-finger-edge of the hands downwards and scoop them out-and-up to above eye level, stretch both arms forwards to the maximum (Figure '2'). Slowly bring them back down the same way, turning the hands over to rest them by the sides.

Repeat 4 times in all, smoothly.

2 'Separate Heaven and Earth'.

This is the second posture. This has pronounced effect on the Spleen, Gall and Stomach. It can aid the digestive functions as well as stretching major and minor side-muscle groups. Therefore regularity will help eliminate risk of gastrointestinal disease or aid in their cure.

THE FORM.
Slowly raise both hands, as before (Figure left). Continue to raise the left hand slowly as high as possible. Simultaneously lower the right hand to behind the right thigh (fingertips outwards on both hands). Stretch the two apart, as though pushing apart the sky and the earth. Look at the upper hand (Figure right).

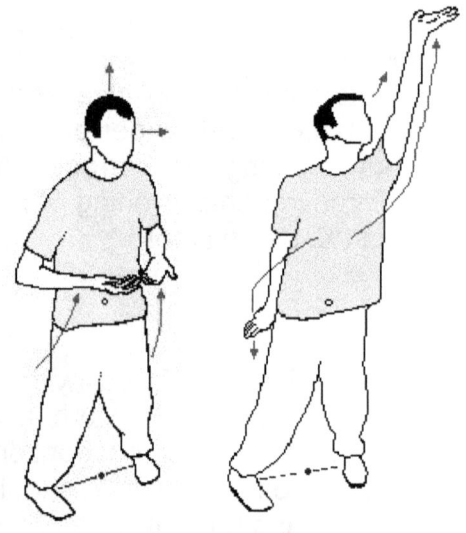

Next, bring them slowly down to the starting position – as in Figure left - and change over, raising the right hand and lowering the left hand.

Do this 4 times each side. Relax to finish, hands by the sides.

3 'Looking Behind You'.

This obviously has a physically more pronounced effect on the neck and head region, although a certain amount of 'massage' is applied to the Kidney area while the muscles of the Spine and torso are also stretched and toned. When turning the head, you are stimulating the muscles of the neck (cervical and vertebra), throat and eyes. Special note may be made to the strengthening of the eye muscles[10], stimulus of the cervical muscles to promote health of the brain and systemic nerves. It

---

[10] Opticians will tell you that the eye muscles are soft tissue and can not be exercised, however, it has long been the belief in TCM that exercises such as this improve the quality of all tissues including the eyes.

is also useful to improve equilibrium in patients with Hypertension and Arteriosclerosis. A noted lessening of mental fatigue may be partly due to a refreshing stimulation of the central nervous system. Considering that the general distribution passage of the nervous system runs along the path of the vertebrae, then it is no surprise that this exercise can have a positive effect on the rest of the body and internal functions.

THE FORM
'Looking Behind You'. Start as in Figure below left. Inhale quietly and deeply without strain.

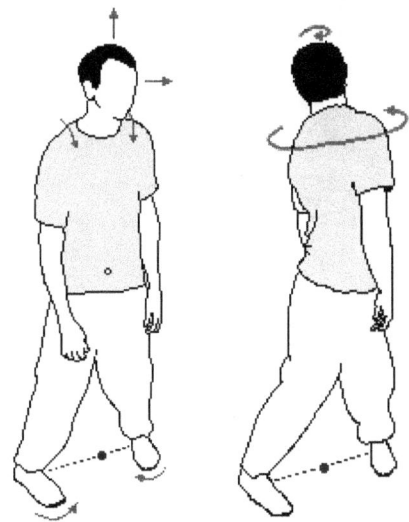

Slowly turn the upper-torso to the left, exhale slowly as you turn. Gently peer over your relaxed shoulders at the floor – approximately forty-five degrees angle (Figure right). This should be felt to put a gentle and comfortable 'squeeze' on the Kidney / Adrenal Gland area, thus helping to rid toxins from the Kidneys and improve the waste elimination processes. The amount by which an individual bends and twists is governed by his or her ability and fitness. Remember never to force a movement, in time and with regular practice flexibility will improve.

Slowly return to the starting posture (left) as you inhale and look straight ahead. Keep weight sinking down. Repeat very slowly and gently 4 times each side.

4 'Riding on Horseback and Drawing the Bow'.

The Chinese health practitioners consider the upper-chest (Thorax) region to be second only in importance to the head. This exercise stretches and expands the chest, enhances the activities of the Lungs and Heart, stretches and tones the muscles in the arms, shoulders and armpit region including Lymph Glands. It is known to assist also in the ridding of pathogenic symptoms resulting from negativity or neglect.

THE FORM
Begin by shifting your weight to your right leg. Step out left with the left foot into the "Riding a Horse" stance. Sink the weight down as low as possible. Bring the hands up to cross in front of

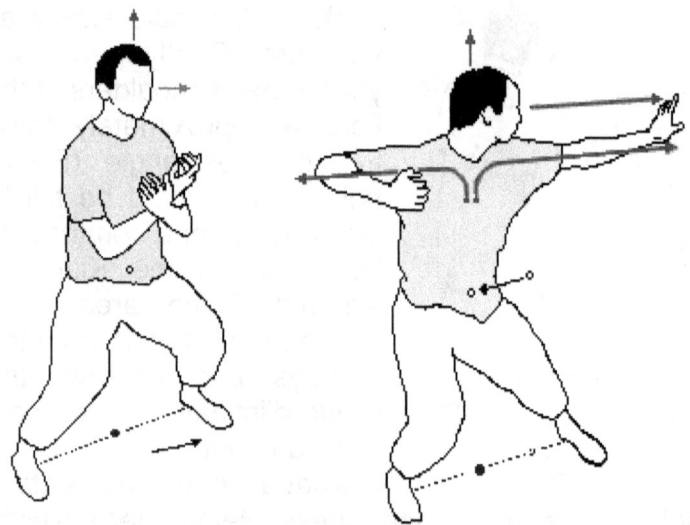

the chest - left hand in front. Look ahead and keep your head aloft (figure on left). Slowly stretch out the left hand with thumb edge towards the ceiling. Stretch the arm out naturally but positively. Simultaneously, pull the right hand back at shoulder level, fingers curled, as though drawing a bowstring. Look at the left index-finger's nail (Figure, right above). At maximum stretch, relax and return to the position as in Figure on left, but this time with the right hand in front. Repeat the 'bow pulling' to the right, exchanging details. Keep the spine straight. Repeat 4 times on each side.   Slide left foot in to end.

5 'Searching The Clouds and Ground'.

This exercise rotates the spine from top-to-tail with the lower 'lumbar' region being the pivotal point. The Chinese say that this exercise 'removes Heart Heat'. 'Heart Heat' has no accurate description in Western medical terms, but it is associated with the symptoms of stress and anxiety in Acupressure, among other things. One point where the intrinsic energy (Qi/Ch'i) can 'block-up' is on the Governor Meridian at the base of the spine. It also translates as being to do with the sympathetic nervous system. A healthy person may be rid of tensions and stress after a rest. Some people do not shed negativity and daily strains quite so easily. In this case there may be a build-up of tension leading to ill health. In summary this exercise rotates the spine, massages the nerves, releases tension and helps the internal functions.

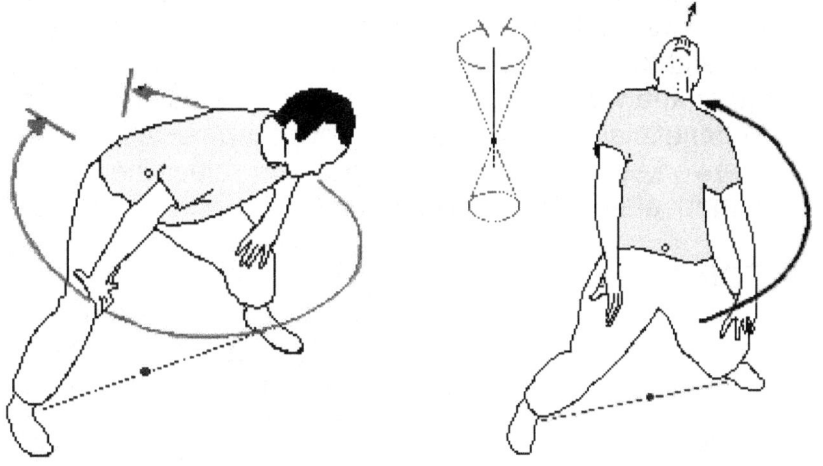

THE FORM (beware of compression of the spine!)
Begin by shifting your body weight to your right leg and inhale. Step out left with the left foot into the "Riding a Horse" stance. Sink the weight down as low as possible. Place the hands on the knees, thumbs and forefingers upwards. Then slowly exhale and lean forward, looking at the ground. Rotate the trunk to the left (Figure on right). Stop before you are leaning back directly, you should be at a slight angle and looking at the sky, inhale and stretch upwards. The spine is pivoting on the axis of the Lumbar Region (see inset diagram) in a dual cone shape.

Rotate back the way you came and look again at the floor as you exhale. Carry on around to the right and repeat the exercise 4 times in each direction.

Notes:
The Discs between the Vertebra can be ruptured if you squeeze them too much. Please see the warning on p.184 regarding the spine in this type of exercise. You are again reminded here of the need to train under the supervision of a properly qualified Teacher who has been shown how this exercise, or ones like it, can be done safely and properly.

6 'Bend to Scoop Water From The Stream'.
This exercise has two halves. In the first sequence we bend from the waist and 'scoop' with our hands. In the later, added sequence we first raise the arms, place the hands on the kidneys and then do the other half. The actions of this exercise strengthen the waist, lumbar, and abdominal regions as well as having beneficial effects on the kidneys themselves. These are the 'overworked' organs that process and reject the unwanted and harmful elements from our bodies.

THE FORM (beware of the spine!)
Start from normal relaxed stance, then raise your hands to abdomen height, as in Figure on left, while raising the Qi. Slowly exhale as you bend the knees and bend forwards, keeping the spine stretched forwards and straight. As you reach your lowest point, extend the hands downwards, as though scooping water from a stream by your feet (Figure on right). Inhale as you stand up and allow the Qi to 'wash down' from the head. Take the hands behind you and perform a Kidney rub, then bring the hands and the Qi up over the

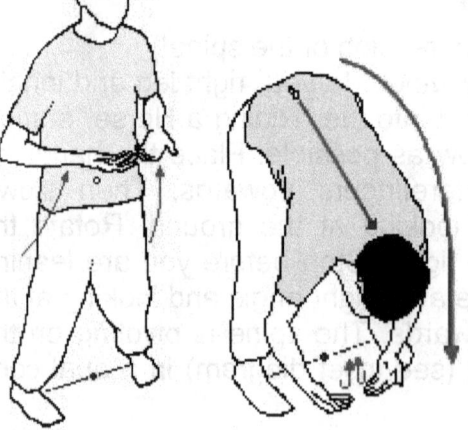

head and back down the front of the body; as in normal 'Qi gathering'. Return to 'centre' before continuing with the next sequence.

Repeat 4 times. Centre and slide your left foot in to finish.

7 Punching Slant-wise and Glaring'.
This exercise increases strength and stimulates the Cerebral Cortex. There are two main variations of this exercise, one internal and one external but in reality they both cross each other's paths. Stretching the first knuckle joints outwards and glaring at the fist with the eyes produces a higher degree of strength and energy.

THE FORM
Begin by shifting your entire weight to your right leg. Step out left with the left foot into the "Riding a Horse" stance. Pull both fists up to your waist as you settle and sink your weight down as low as possible. Avoid tension: Keep the shoulders relaxed, chest concave, back and head upright and your eyes gazing straight ahead (Figure on left). Slowly, punch the left fist outward at a 45 degree outward-and-upwards angle. Keep the head stretched up and the lower spine sunk down and straight. Glare your eyes at the outstretched fist (Figure on right). Slowly relax the arm as you return to the starting posture.

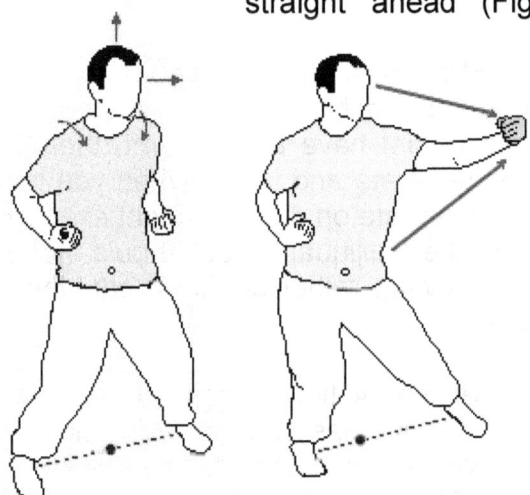

Repeat this exercise 4 times with each arm. Pull in the left foot to finish.

8 Stand on Tip-Toe and Shake'.

This may be done up to eight times, regardless of how many repetitions you made of the others. This gently shakes the internal organs back into place and relaxes. It is an ideal way of finishing (closing) and should be followed by a short period of standing quietly whilst concentrating on the Dantian/Tan T'ien point just below the navel.

THE FORM

Starting posture for this is as in Figure 'A'. Stand-up on tip-toes (and ball-of-foot) until you feel as though lifted to full stretch by a thread attached to the top of the head. Inhale as you do this (Figure '12'). Let the breath escape naturally as you suddenly 'release', dropping the heels to within one centimetre of the floor *. Repeat 8 times.

* Important: Do not let the heels 'bump' on the floor as this causes jolting of the spine which is not healthy. The idea is to gently shake the internal organs into place and 'vibrate' them and the nervous systems in a gentle and caring manner.

The Eight Strands of Brocade should be done every day to achieve best results. Its movements at first have to be learnt, therefore they will be separate and jerky. When you have learnt them you should concentrate on doing all eight exercises smoothly and joined up, like Taijiquan. You should not be tense when stretching or moving, rather be like a cat when it stretches, lithe and relaxed.

After initially doing the exercises 4 times each on each side, aim to do more. Increase it to 8 times each on each side and do the whole set. When your stamina allows, you can do the whole set more than once. Always do the whole set and do not just take out one or two of your favourites as this may cause imbalanced exercise and will not do you so much good as originally intended.

The Role of Pa Tuan Chin in Exercise

In Europe most people tend to think of exercise as one or more of the following: walking, weight lifting, jogging, aerobics or dance based exercise and circuit training. In recent years the Box-exercise and yoga systems have also become fairly well known, although usually by those who go to modern fitness emporiums. In most of Europe exercise has not changes that much since the end of Victorian times, there have just been a few changes to the equipment used as well as medical advances in recognising the importance of posture or other effects on the body, most importantly using exercise for better health and healing.

In China exercise has not changed that much either over a hundred years or so. The reasons for this are different. China has a longer history than Great Britain and longer than most European countries too. Some older European countries though have never had a proper system of exercise, or anything beyond the local cultural dance routine. The Chinese are an inquisitive race. China has been responsible for the invention of most things which the vast majority of people worldwide take for granted nowadays, like: Paper, printing, banknotes, gunpowder, silk and weaving, kites, armoured ships, rockets, guns, Aerial warfare, typewriters, irrigation, clocks, etcetera, etcetera. Surprised?

The Chinese are a great nation of discoverers and inventors. Elsewhere in this book you will read about two of the greatest men who ever lived, Dr. Hua To and "The Yellow Emperor " Huang Ti. If children in schools in the UK and Europe were taught accurate history as well as history including the Chinese past and contributions to civilised society then perhaps we would see a change of values in our own cultures for the better. Children would realise that the Chinese Arts have much to offer the West and perhaps take a different approach to exercise and medicine as well as invention.

It has to be said that modern western exercise is still lacking. No matter how trendy the gym or fitness warehouse you go to you will see, if you know what to look for, that the exercise classes are struggling to provide good quality exercise. Many exercise instructors "borrow" ideas from Indian or Chinese exercise systems like Yoga, Pranayama, Taijiquan or Taoist Yoga. Take Pilates, for instance, this it seems is a mixture of Indian Yoga with a little Chinese influence. Most fitness clubs now offer what they call 'Core Stability' exercises. These are blatantly core principles of Taijiquan (T'ai Chi Ch'uan) in the main - posture and relaxation - with a somewhat liberal, in some cases, helping of personal translation by budding exercise and fitness instructors.

Anyone who has been teaching exercise conscientiously over the past twenty or more years with an eye on safety and common sense will see that the exercise industry, as they call it, is struggling to keep up with itself. This struggle is born of their own existence because they all want to do something different which attracts new members; read as 'new money', approximately £30 - £60 per person monthly (2009 Average).

Baduanjin (Pa T'uan Chin) is a highly developed form of exercise which has roots going back many hundreds of years. It has connections with other forms or methods of Chinese physical culture, including Taijiquan and Daoist K'ai Men Yoga. It is hard to say whether Baduanjin started out as Qigong or a stretch based exercise system, maybe both. What we do know is that it has developed and changed over the years, not always for the better, as with most things. On occasion it seems that an individual has taken the basic concepts of Baduanjin and reworked it to suit themselves or some other purpose; unknown. Sometimes these reworked exercises may be undertaken with the mind to make it more difficult, therefore making the performer look almost superhuman compared to those not able to do some of the contortions. Perhaps they just wanted to make the exercises more difficult as a challenge, a step towards super-yogic flexibility, or something. The moral here is that not all forms of exercise are what they seem or indeed necessary. Difficult exercises may also be harmful to the body. This is why a thoughtfully developed standardised form is needed with clearly defined guidelines for instructors.

Baduanjin's role is simple. It is an extremely well designed form of eight exercises which can help balance and maintain the human body. I feel almost certain that the original concept must have been to open up the joints, stretch the muscles and ligaments, open the energy channels and generally maintain one's health with minimum fuss, bother, space or equipment. If this is true then the original developer must have been a truly great scientist.

In modern society, as stated above, we lack a steady exercise method as well as a well developed, tried, tested and proved system. Taijiquan is having a great effect on many people but there is a problem with this in so much as there are many different styles of Taijiquan. There is Chen, with its foot stamping and vigorous waist turning – a great Martial Art but hardly suitable for the frail or unfit - then there is Yang Style with its wide steps and 'large frame' movements (though I am told that there are too many people practising too many variations, making it difficult to learn as you travel, and some of the stances could provide potential danger to the knees if done incorrectly. There are also Wu/Hao, Wu and Lee and Sun Family styles, all with some similarities. These are all classic and worthwhile styles of Taijiquan but can not be classified as 'general exercise', even though they are all very beneficial for health and fitness.

Baduanjin offers a more suitable option. As it stretches, tones, opens the channels for Ch'i to flow it could be said that it offers not only a good daily routine to us all but could act as a 'gateway' into exercise for the unfit, an excellent stretching routine for the already fit and indeed a gateway to Taijiquan. A brilliant warm up routine for sports men or women done in a more rigorous manner, and a relaxing set at that for those who are suffering from tension and stress. It also has another function, that of Qigong / Ch'i Kung exercise of course, as it opens up the energy channels (meridians) really well and helps strengthen the flow of bioenergy (Ch'i) throughout the body. There is no other simple exercise routine that I know of which does all of this and can be practised so easily by so many. Baduanjin is the ideal starter and compliment to any Martial Art, Sports, Taijiquan practice or as a stand alone exercise program[11]. Not forgetting that this is the New Standardised Set as well and that it has been developed and taught with safety and variation built in; adaptability. This puts it in the elemental class of Water, for water can adapt to any shape or environment.

In our "modern" (I am smiling wryly when writing that word) society Baduanjin has a special place. In our society we have much illness and imbalance. This is because we have the wrong values when it comes to food and living in general. Our bodies are constantly polluted with junk food, fumes, chemicals and residue fall-out from the atmosphere.

Many medical practitioners of the Orthodox system (as practised in hospitals and GP's surgeries) are now looking towards T'ai Chi Ch'uan as a gentle exercise which can cure many imbalances and help fight many common illnesses, like arthritis, for example. The famous Dr. Paul Lam has developed the 12 Step Sun Style Form for Arthritis sufferers. Pa Tuan Chin is also suitable for arthritis sufferers, if adjusted according to condition, as well as many other ailments. It can be taken up by almost anyone, including those who can not stand, to enhance the quality of their health.

Pa Tuan Chin is one of those exercise systems which has been overlooked, until now, by the West and is not only comparable to T'ai Chi Ch'uan but is far more flexible or adaptable. It is my hope that the UK and European medical systems will take this flexible exercise system on board and give it time and room for its full potential to be realised. As an instructor you could play an active part in this development.

---

[11]Footnote 1: I use the American spelling of program as the English "programme" is a bit loquacious.

REGISTERED TTT BADUANJIN INSTRUCTORS:
(*Strictly No Advertising Calls, Spam Email or Sales)

Location:	UK, Norfolk. HQ & Instructor Training (see p.220)*
Open to:	Teacher Training / Medical Staff / Therapists / Etc.
Location:	**London and Kent**
Name:	Dr. Mark Green
Contact:	*greentaichi@yahoo.co.uk / 07976-969868
Location:	**UK, East Grinstead.**
Name:	Shih-fu Bill Bostock
Open to:	Private Lessons / Small Groups.
Contact:	*Tel. 01342-328753 / Fax. 0870-1623904. E-mail bill@bostock.com
Mail:	*Kamon Martial Art Federation c/o 31 The Old Convent, East Grinstead, West Sussex, RH19 3RS
Location:	**UK, North Norfolk.**
Name:	Shih-fu F. Lee (Tiandidao).
Open to:	Local Day Classes, Lectures: e.g. W.I., Rotary Club, etc.
Contact:	*Tel. 01263-513866
Other:	Tai Chi for Health, Qigong, Trad. Taijiquan & Yang.
Location:	**UK, Norfolk & Elsewhere.**
Name:	Dr. William Hughes. / Traumacare Network.
Open to:	Hospital Staff Training / Disabled / Elderly / Traumatised Individuals.
Contact:	*Tel. 01603-503845 / Fax. 01603-502272
Mail:	Traumacare Network, The Coach House, Church Avenue, Norwich NR2 2AQ, England.
Location:	**UK, East Sussex / Hastings & St. Leonards.**

Name:	Shih-fu Nick O'Shaughnessy
Open to:	Elderly / Disabled / Children / Substance Misuse / +
Contact:	*Tel. 07882-730255 / info@healthtaichi.co.uk
Other:	Qigong & Baduanjin / Chen Man Ching Taijiquan / Tai Chi for Arthritis .
Location:	**UK, Suffolk / Lowestoft area.**
Name:	Shih-fu Erik Tyler (Tiandidao)
Open to:	Community / Health Care.
Contact:	*07906-169221
Location:	**UK, West Scotland /**
Name:	Johnny Glover.
Open to:	General / Community / Groups / Health Care.
Contact:	01776704994 / johnny@jgyoga.co.uk
Mail:	JGYoga, 84 Eastwood Avenue, Stranraer, Wigtownshire, Scotland DG9 8DT
Location:	**Ireland / Cork area.**
Name:	David Boyle – Rochestown Qigong Centre.
Open to:	Community (Also Registered in Chinese Medicine)
Contact:	00353-(0)87-873-0761 / dchiboyle@hotmail.com
Mail:	Rochestown Physical Therapy and Acupuncture Clinic, Rochestown, Cork, Ireland.
Location:	**UK, Surrey / Guildford.**
Name:	Tanya Pritchard
Open to:	Community
Contact:	07721-379561 (Mobile)

Personal Notes and findings on Qigong:

Name:_____Dates:_____

The Author's Background

Professor Mike Symonds.
Chief Instructor and Founder of
T'IEN TI TAO CH'UAN-SHU P'AI.

The only Personal Invite student (being a non-member) to Teacher's Training 'Choi Kung' – 1975 to 1980 – of the late Grandmaster Soo, Clifford Chee. Founder and head of the International Taoist Arts Association (ITAA).
& Chinese Cultural Arts Association (CCAA).

East Anglian Representative for AMA (Kung Fu) c.1980-85.

East Anglian Ambassador for BKPA (UK branch of ICKF).
c.1985 to 1989.

Instructor in chief, British Association for Chinese Arts (c. 1995 to 2000).

C.E.O. of the Martial Arts & Fitness Coach UK/EU
www.mafcuk.org (2001 to   )

STUDIES INCLUDE:
Buddhist Philosophy, Tibetan Buddhism, Sufi Philosophy, Christianity, Taoist Philosophy, Social Behaviour & Community.
Karate, Kempo, Chinese Martial Arts/Fighting Systems/History/Theory and Principles.
Taoist K'ai Men (Open Gates) Yoga, Hatha Yoga to Pranayama, Buddhist Yoga.
Taoist Ch'ang Ming (Long Life) Diet, Nutrition, Herbs (Western).
Taoist Chi Kung – plus some Confucian and Buddhist.
Taoist Health & Healing Arts (Acupressure, massage, etc.)
T'ai Chi Ch'uan & Dr. Paul Lam's adapted Sun Style Tai Chi for Arthritis.
Meditations and Special Exercises for Spiritual Advancement and Protection.

PERSONAL BACKGROUND:
Practised "Chinese Shadow Boxing" since early childhood informally. Took up serious study in mid-to-late sixties alongside philosophies and other studies.

T'IEN TI TAO© ACADEMY

Chief Instructor:
Shih-fu Mike Symonds.
35 years teaching and coaching experience (at 2009).

National and International Students.

Please contact:
www.Tai-Chi-Kungfu.com
or www.TTTkungfu.com

E-mail:
enquiries@TTTkungfu.com

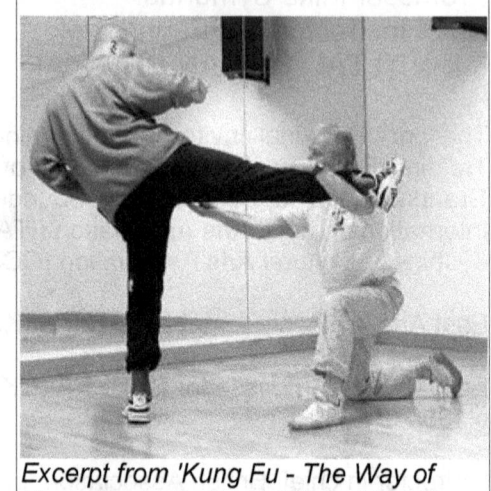

Excerpt from 'Kung Fu - The Way of Heaven and Earth' (published by Life Force UK)

Strictly No Spam; Spam or unrequested Junk e-mails are reported to ISP's, Government Bodies, Criminal Investigation Units, etcetera.

ENQUIRIES ABOUT REGULAR CLASSES or COURSES:
PA TUAN CHIN - T'AI CHI CH'UAN – TAOIST KUNG FU & THERAPIES - TAOIST YOGA – StressBusta™ - TAI CHI for HEALTH, WOMEN'S 'Wild Rose' SELF-DEFENCE - + MORE.

All Content herein, Images (except those from ancient Chinese wood-block prints), Forms and Exercise Sets, Illustrations, ideas and phrases are Copyright. For permission to reproduce in part for reviews, news or other media presentations, please apply in good time to the above e-mail address stating your name, company and reasons and we will reply. Thank you.

OTHER BOOKS AVAILABLE BY THE SAME AUTHOR

Kung Fu – The Way of Heaven & Earth.
This book includes the most accurate potted history of Chinese Martial Arts development to date, plus the history of the famous Wu Tang ("Wudang") Mountains in China's heartlands, the home of Taoism. There is a useful section detailing basic cautions in exercising, especially in Martial Arts (applicable to all styles) as well as a comprehensive and mind expanding article written about Forms ("Dalu") and Form Practice.

Also included are the first three syllabus sections of Tiandidao which not only serve to help new students get a stronger foundation but also show what a well structured and carefully thought out system this is. Tiandidao is the first and only system of Traditional Chinese Martial Arts to have been developed by a Westerner, then tested and accepted by the largest Traditional Chinese Martial Arts group in the world and accepted as "Genuine traditional Chinese Arts" where one Old Master apparently commented, "It's probably more traditional than most traditional systems!"

Tai Chi Diet: food for life
(Taoist Ch'ang Ming/Long Life Diet)
Description: For many centuries the Chinese Taoists have known the secrets of balanced diet and good health. Foods are like medicine or poison, like herbs (another form of food) they can heal or make ill. Learn how to detect illness or imbalance, how to correct your diet and live longer with more energy. Special needs section covers common illnesses like cancer, migraines, hypoglycaemia, rheumatism and more.

The Martial Arts & Fitness Instructor's *Invaluable* Guide.
This book was first released in 2002 as a free gift for new members of Martial Arts & Fitness Coach UK (www.mafcuk.org), but is now undergoing updates and extra content with lots of useful information.

(Available through: www.Life-Force-publishing.co.uk or any International book seller source including on-line book sellers)

www.ingramcontent.com/pod-product-compliance
Lightning Source LLC
Chambersburg PA
CBHW050142170426
43197CB00011B/1935